Healing by Intent

A Medical Memoir

John Graham-Pole

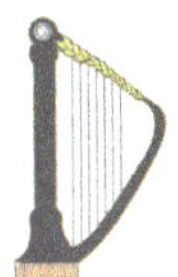

HARP Publishing
The People's Press
Clydesdale, Nova Scotia
Canada

HARP Publishing The People's Press
216 Clydesdale Road
Clydesdale, Nova Scotia
Canada B2G 2K9

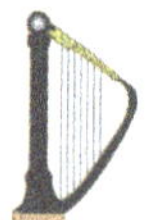

www.harppublishing.ca

harppeoplespress@gmail.com

tel# 902.863.0396

Catalogue-in-Publication data is on file with Library and Archives Canada

ISBN: 978-0-9938295-8-1

Graphic design: Cathy Lin
Cover Art: Sara Avmaat

The Circle of Abundance Indigenous Program, Coady International Institute, St. Francis Xavier University: https://coady.stfx.ca/circle-of-abundance; and David Suzuki Foundation (one nature): https://davidsuzuki.org will receive 20% of all sales, distributed equally.

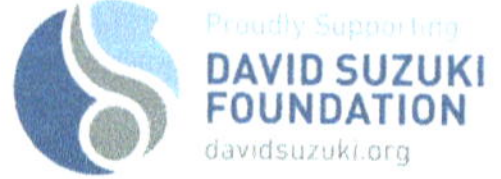

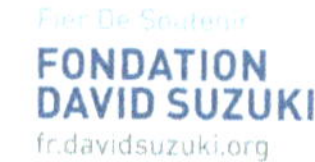

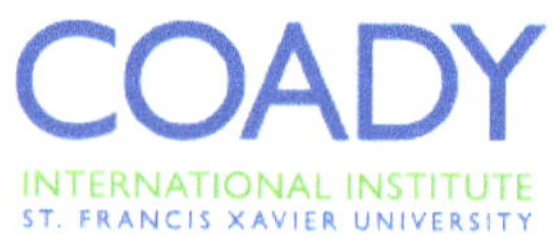

Also by John Graham-Pole

Non-Hodgkin's Lymphoma
Illness and the Art of Creative Self-Expression
Physical
On Wings of Spirit (Co-Authored)
Quick: A Pediatrician's Illustrated Poetry
The Arts & Health (Co-Authored)
Journeys with a Thousand Heroes
The People's Photo Album (Co-Authored)
The Heroes Trilogy:

- Blood Work
- A Boy and his Soul
- Songlines

Praise for Healing by Intent

Thank you for the privilege of reviewing your second medical memoir. The key messages highlight important truths for both medical colleagues and the public. Easy to read, interspersed with humour through even the most difficult times, often filled with hope. There are moments of absolute clinical clarity that are often hard but always necessary. The hand that guides us is always gentle, caring, memorable.

Three highlights: children as patients—always a heartwarming and often humbling experience; coping with death—a frequent visitor when cancer has been your specialty; being at peace with your role—enabling you to care in profound ways for your patients and their families.

Rosie Richardson, MBBS, Consultant Paediatrician, Cornwall, UK

Healing By Intent lifts the veil into the intimate interactions between doctor and patient. Dr. Graham-Pole offers a glimpse into the subtle dance of learning and healing for both doctor and patient. His ability to reach the essential human connection in his relationships with children with cancer and to let the story of those connections unfold is brilliantly captured in this memoir. His gentleness and kindness with patients are a master class in the wisdom he has gained from many years of listening to the stories of these remarkable young people. John is a man of quiet courage and deep compassion, and in this book he does one of the things he does best: opening the path for us to become better caregivers through his storytelling and his kindness.

Anne Rossi, MD, Pediatric Hematologist and Oncologist,
Maine, USA

Dr. Graham-Pole's splendidly crafted memoir is much more than an autobiography. It may be read straight through as you would read any regular memoir; but it may also be read a chapter at a time, picking almost any at random. Each chapter is its own magnificent tribute to the heroic children who were his patients, their families, his colleagues, his friends, and the author himself as he goes about doing good, bringing hope and humour and healing to seemingly hopeless situations.

Readers will find starkly honest accounts of his childhood, adolescence and years of training to become a specialist in treating childhood cancers. His lyrical prose is like several strokes of an artist's brush—delicate, soft, hard, intense, delicate once more. The canvas of his work is brilliant, intimate, breathtaking—as if the curtains were peeled back for the privilege of peering into his very soul.

Francis Christian, MD, FRCSEd, FRCSC, Consultant Surgeon,
Saskatoon, Saskatchewan

As a pediatric oncologist with a gift for storytelling, John Graham-Pole has shared stories depicting the diversity in human experiences related to sickness, recovery, and death. His vignettes focus on the meaning of healing, revealing its complexity along several dimensions including despair and hope, fragility and strength, sadness and humour. These stories about young patients and their families unveil human strength, in spirit if not always in body. They also remind us of the important role of caregivers in fostering physical, psychological, and spiritual healing.

Doris Gillis, PhD, Professor of Nutrition, St. Francis Xavier University,
Antigonish, Nova Scotia

This book should be on the reading list of any young person considering a career in medicine. Immensely readable and extraordinarily frank, Dr. Graham-Pole has drawn upon his forty years as a children's oncologist to describe the messages children and their families have given him about living and coping with long term medical conditions—many fatal—and the lessons he has been privileged to learn. Events and conversations are re-constructed from contemporaneous notes and conversations into a series of reflective stories. Each one reveals the fears and hopes of children and their parents, but also how the theory underlying medical practise is only a part of what is needed if a doctor is to provide the in-depth care such situations demand.

Whilst courage and love shine through each story, John conveys the contribution that honesty, self-evaluation, patience, shared understanding, and sometimes silence, play in good care for both doctor and patient. These are lessons learnt in practise, not always ranked high enough or given sufficient attention in a medical curriculum densely packed with academic knowledge to be learnt. Yet these lessons underpin so much of what can be great medical care.

Every story is exciting and unsettling. The benefit of compassion and understanding given by the doctor is very evident, but so is the reward felt from gaining ever deeper insight into human nature. Young and aspiring doctors, please note!

Diane Smyth, MD, FRCP, Consultant Pediatric Neurologist, London, UK

Once again, Dr. Graham-Pole shares his rich life experiences caring for and walking beside children living and dying with cancer. John's vivid and poignant story telling reminds us that medical science may often cure disease but it is the healing arts that touch our common humanity—offering meaning and relieving suffering of families living through these life-changing ordeals.

Phillip Cooper, MD, Palliative Care Physician,
Oncology Associate, and Anglican Postulant, Antigonish, Nova Scotia

I would recommend this memoir as an account of an English childhood long past, but more importantly as an insight into the bravery of families with challenging illness and their need for an empathic physician who encourages space for humour. The author's use of language is accessible to all. The cast become real people in a few sentences, heart-breaking at times. I particularly liked the times when medical personnel fell short of humanity. Paediatrics is rarely about a single patient, with parents, siblings, grandparents, friends and pets being crucial to the picture.

Susan Thompson, MBBS, Consultant Paediatrician, UK

Healing by Intent is ravishing, hopeful, and inspirational! This book is a must-read for health care professionals who work towards intentionally changing people's lives. John Graham-Pole's wise and thoughtful memoir enables health care professionals and others to see life as it is, if we are to move forward on the many challenges people face. Only through a symbiosis of healing by intent can we enable the social changes we all need.

Jubanti Toppo, Social Worker, Adult Educator,
Former UNCSW Delegate for Canada

John Graham-Pole has lived an extraordinary life and has an equally extraordinary ability to translate his experiences into poetry on the page. In *Healing by Intent*, his second memoir surveying his forty-year career as a physician, he takes us on a journey from the first physical he administered at St Bartholomew's Hospital in London back in 1963 on the frail but feisty (and decidedly not pregnant) Mrs. Lovell, through to his final years as a member of the pediatric faculty at the University of Florida—all told through short-story vignettes featuring a vivid cast of characters, young and old.

Although he considers his recollections to stem from what he calls "messy" memories, his stories and the dialog that drives them feel crisp, clear, and full of living reality. He extracts grace and humour from moments of tragedy—a testament to his devotion to the power of medicine and the wisdom of the Quaker faith, which brought him strength in unfathomably sad and desperate situations. You can feel his kindness and gentle demeanor in the ways he lovingly describes patients, friends, and the many people he encountered in his career as a healer.

This is a book filled with uplifting stories of young lives saved (some through music as much as medicine) and sad stories of young lives lost; but you will not be left with sadness in your heart. You will finish this book with a renewed faith in the good of humanity and wonder at the power of one person to leave such a striking legacy of peace in his wake.

Justin Gregg, PhD,
Author, Editor, Actor

I was fortunate to work with John Graham-Pole for much of his forty-year career in medicine, and I've seen how he heals himself and others through loving kindness, humour, empathy. and love. *Healing by Intent* recounts the stories by which he does this healing. Each chapter of this beautiful memoir is a story from his personal or professional life. Some of the stories recount his personal journey, but most are stories of his heroes—those children with cancer who bore their disease with dignity and grace and who helped him to heal himself and others.

He shows us how he was comforted by comforting, how his inner resources and his Quaker faith helped him through difficult times, and how the children inspired him. In my favourite story—"Origin of an Epidemic"—he recounts the physical, psychological, legal and ethical dilemmas of those young heroes with hemophilia affected by HIV in the first years of this pandemic. Earlier, John tells us that "everyone has a story, everyone is a story," and he offers proof of this in his beautiful, authentic collection of stories from his personal and professional life.

Paulette Mehta, MD, MPH, Professor of Hematology & Oncology;
Poetry Editor, "Medicine and Meaning", University of Arkansas for Medical Sciences

This is an inspirational book which should be on the reading list of all medical students and young doctors.

The early chapters cover the problems facing a young boy who has lost his mother from cancer at an early age. John experiences different social backgrounds from the working class north to the stockbroker belt of the southeast of England. There is internal conflict between the aggressive captain of the boxing team and the student of the classics. The book traces his path through medical school into the emotionally challenging field of paediatric oncology. There are vivid accounts of some of his cases which give us understanding of paediatric cancers and blood disorders.

Fundamental to the book is John's quest to find the answer to coping with seriously ill children, helped by his spirituality and Quaker faith. Medical science has made great advances, but the contribution of art, music and humour are equally important in the healing process. I am reminded of Voltaire: "The art of medicine consists in amusing the patient while nature cures the disease."

John Roger Boston, BA. MB. B.Chir. FRCS (Eng)

Dr. Graham-Pole's humility in knowing that a higher being is ultimately responsible for our healing is immeasurable. The combination of acquired knowledge, hard work, and humility is characteristic of the greatest of physicians.

The artistic descriptions of his childhood made me time-travel, as well as causing me to feel the emotion of each patient interaction. This is story telling at its finest. The collection of individual stories gives a glimpse into the doctor-patient relationship that is so cherished by the author. As the sibling of someone who had cancer as a young child and whom Dr. Graham-Pole treated, this memoir reminded me of my family's own journey and renewed my faith in God, in medicine, and in humanity.

Bonnie Skinner
Sister of a child with cancer and bone marrow transplant donor

John Graham-Pole is a compelling storyteller. As with his previous book, *Journeys With A Thousand Heroes*, the main focus of the stories in *Healing by Intent* is the lessons learned in communication, community and relationship, from children, families, and healthcare colleagues. In addition to the stories, the opening essay offers us reflections on healing in its deepest sense. Additionally, John offers us a glimpse into how Quaker worship intertwines with his experience as a pediatric oncologist to inculcate a deep respect for silent witness and deep listening.

If you don't want to cry, don't read this book. If you don't want to smile through the tears, don't read this book.

Sara Avmaat
Artist and Physiotherapist

"Everyone has a story; everyone is a story." A gifted storyteller, John Graham-Pole sensitively relates his own story—an authentic and intimate journey, with childhood heartaches balanced by appreciation for the gift of lessons learned and opportunities grasped along the way.

As I pored through the stories, a favorite line from "Bone Marrow Tale"—a poem John wrote two decades ago to comfort a young pediatric fellow after her night with a dying child—kept coming to mind: "not much frightens you, proficient lover of hurting humans." So true for John as well. In *Healing with Intent*, his thoughts and questionings reveal a continuing exploration of a lifetime of loving service to the youngest of those hurting humans among us.

Judy Rollins, PhD, RN, Adjunct Assistant Professor,
Family Medicine and Pediatrics, Georgetown University, Washington, DC.

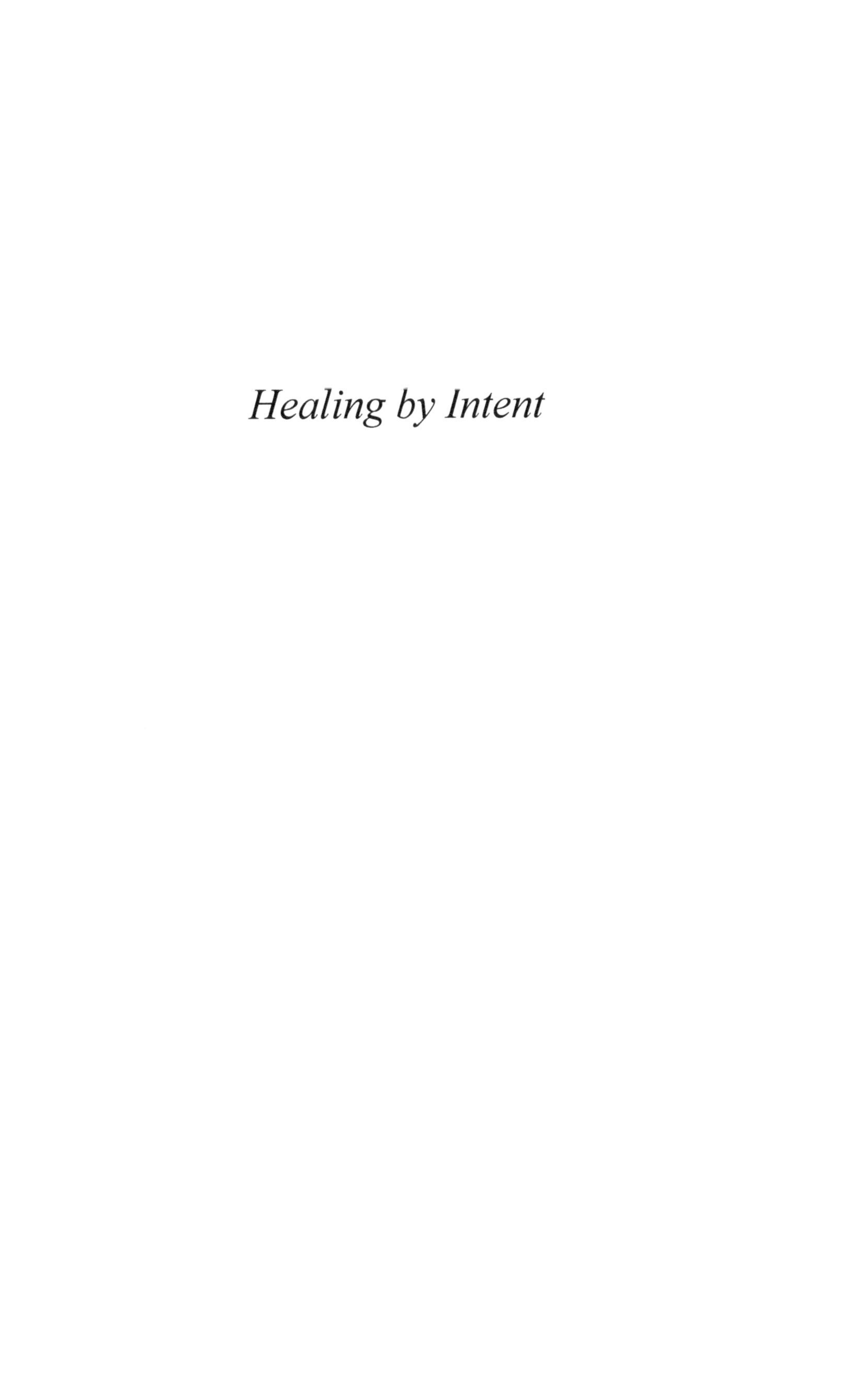

Healing by Intent

Contents

Permissions

Several of these essays have been published in earlier forms and are reproduced here with the permission of the respective journal editors:

The Surgeon	Hektoen, 2011
First Physical	Ars Medica, 2015
More Encounters with Surgeons	Journal of Surgical Humanities, 2017
Origin of an Epidemic	Medical Literary Messenger, 2018
Connective Tissue	Medicine and Meaning, 2021
Midder	Blood and Thunder, 2021
Twins	Hektoen, 2021

Prologue

The art of medicine consists in amusing the patient while nature cures the disease.

Voltaire

When God wants an important thing done, he simply has a tiny baby born, perhaps in a very humble home of a very humble mother.

Marian Wright Edelman

Edith was the ward clerk on our bone marrow transplant unit where I worked as a pediatric oncologist in the University of Florida's Shands Hospital. I co-directed the unit with Alan, a medical oncologist, and when we opened the six-bedded unit in 1982, we decided we would share the beds equally: three for adults and three for children. Edith carried out the endless clerical and administrative duties, checking patients in and out of the unit, filing their paperwork, coordinating their assignments with the nurses and doctors. Only later did I find out that this graceful black woman had raised a large family, and now was putting herself through seminary to become a Baptist minister.

Edith was core to the efficient running of the unit, hence her front seat at the nurses' station. When I was the attending physician for the month, I would start out every day wrapped in Edith's arms for a lingering hug. In memory she was always the hugger and I the huggee; she was the mom I hadn't had since I was twelve. As our friendship deepened, she would share "just-between-you-and-me" stories. This is how I came to learn that our patients and their families shared more intimate moments with Edith than they ever would with their doctors. And how I came to see a larger meaning to the word, *healing*. That healing embraces listening, loving witness, and prayerful intent.

Healing has its origin in wounds—physical, psychological, spiritual—often all three interwoven. Our bodily wounds heal either by first—often called primary—or by secondary intent. First intent leaves no tissue loss so there is no scar, or only a skinny one. Second intent means the wound's edges are too far apart to come together cleanly. Healing takes longer and leaves a lasting and visible scar. Either way, it's miraculous. This is the *intent*—conscious or otherwise—of both wounded ones and those who tend to their wounds: to heal.

There is no need—no place—for healing where there is no wound. Perhaps it's no accident that the French word for wound is *blessure*. We are all blessed, like it or not, with wounds. Wounds to our bodies, our minds, our spirits. We live through healing from our earliest childhood; and as children most of our wounds are healed with a loving touch, a kiss to make it better, a murmur of maternal lullaby. But some we carry with us as we grow; perhaps retain them for whole lifetimes. It is in our human nature to turn our wounds into stories, hoping—awarely or unawarely—that we will find another to tell our stories to. Edith our ward clerk knew she had found her life calling: to be a listener—a loving witness—as our patients and their families came to her with their stories. Her attentive ear set them on their paths towards healing.

I believe that more healing took place at Edith's desk in the front of the nurses' station than in any of our isolation rooms. Though I very much doubt the hospital administrators who hired Edith to clerk our bone marrow unit foresaw her role as a healing witness, and she herself would never have spoken of herself as a healer. If anything, she reserved that word for the doctors and nursing staff. We health workers do sometimes fall into the trap of seeing ourselves as healers. But to heal is an *intransitive* verb: when wounded, we do our own healing, or strive to—it's not for others to heal us. Labelling as a healer any doctor or nurse, social worker or psychologist who tends to our physical or emotional wounds, is a misnomer. A rather arrogant one, actually. Benjamin Franklin got it right: "God does the healing and the doctor takes the fee."

Here's another misnomer, or at best a very narrow description. Merriam-Webster defines the word *placebo* as "an inert or innocuous substance used especially in controlled experiments testing the efficacy of another substance." It pays not even lip service to the caregiver's *attention* and *intention* as being such vital placebos. A loving caregiver can feed a patient an inactive placebo-pill, disclose to them that its ingredients are totally inert, yet still witness a measure of healing in their patient. Is this the effect of the pill—something pharmacologists haven't yet been able to detect and analyze? Or is it simply the loving intent of the caregiver who administered it? Is it healing by intent?

I spent forty years caring for young people with cancer. The thousands of children who came to me over my forty years as a doctor were all badly wounded. The wounds of cancer run deep—and cancer is a family's illness. In my early years in medicine—the 1960s and 1970's—most of those children never made it to adulthood. It was only a few years earlier—in 1947—that Dr. Sidney Farber, a pathologist at Boston Children's Hospital, injected the world's first known dose of chemotherapy into the blood of two-year-old Robert Sandler. It was an antifolate drug called aminopterin. His pediatrician colleagues had already shunned him, christening him "doctor of the dead." Farber had earned that label the previous year by conducting a seemingly outlandish experiment. Knowing pregnant women and malnourished children quite often developed a specific anemia caused by folic acid deficiency, he had tested the effect of folic acid on several children with leukemia. The effect was to immediately accelerate their leukemia and even further shorten their lives.

But in Dr. Farber's words, "The 325,000 patients with cancer who are going to die this year cannot wait for great progress in the cure of cancer, for us to have the full solutions to the problems of basic research." In the face of mounting opposition, he went ahead with his reverse experiment—and by New Year's Eve Robert Sandler's leukemia had disappeared. The chemical war on cancer was launched.

But consistent cures for cancer through the use of chemotherapy were several decades in the future. So why were these babies and children and teenagers put on this earth for so short a time? To bless their moms and dads with such joy—only to have to give them up. To give them back. Spending my working life at the bedsides of these deathly ill children, I came to realize that they were my teachers. I watched them experience life's particularities more fully and richly than I ever had, who had submerged my primal memories since my adolescence. So children gave me back much more than I could ever give them—joy in fleeting moments, laughter, valour, disarming candour. They were rarely mournful or intimidated—and if they were, they were quick to let me know why.

I wrote this sonnet as a requiem to these many children who have come and gone so soon.

We offer the oblation of our tears,
as time begins to soften loss's bite;
then laugh, like we did in the springtime of our years,
to the sounds of your music echoed on our night,
moderato cantabile tumbling to our hearth,
as you rap out rhythms on beams of mother moon,
cappricio melodies lighting on the earth,
dancing *bachatas* on the arm of songbird sun.

We hear through the fading light the schoolroom bell,
a *decrescendo* resonance on the breeze,
that beckons you welcome with its whispered knell
to roam at large in celestial childhood fields,
sounding out your tempos till, earth's *etude* done,
you tiptoe *piano* to the arms of the waiting sun.

There is no simple answer to the question of why many of us are destined to live longer and longer lives, while many of those I cared for were granted such terribly short ones. Many suffered from seemingly identical cancers, and by the conventions of modern medicine we grouped them together to receive identical treatment protocols. So why did some make it and others not? Why could my drugs cure some children but not others? It may be logical to categorize those with seemingly identical diseases under one treatment umbrella, but each one of them was of course unique. They all had different stories to tell; they all *were* different stories.

Robert Fulghum in *All I Ever Needed to Know I Learned in Kindergarten* describes the Storyteller's Creed: *imagination, myth, dreams, hope,* and *love* are more powerful than *knowledge, facts, experience, grief,* and *death.* The stories I heard at countless bedsides were decidedly not the ones I overhear at the supermarket check-out line. Those bedside conversations helped build for me, and I hope for the children too, dreams of hope and love.

I wrote my earlier memoir, *Journeys with a Thousand Heroes*: *A Child Oncologist's Story,* as a chronicle of a life in medicine, starting with my mother's death when I was twelve and ending with my retirement fifty-three years later. One of the benefits of aging is that you have time to remember, and to reflect. I found myself recalling more stories from my life as a caregiver, and I began to look for what was *healing* in them. Healing for the children, even those who died, healing for their loved ones, healing for me. Or perhaps all three.

Fourteen-year-old Dan died after his leukemia had resisted all our efforts to control it. I had escorted the gurney that took him from our pediatric ward to the intensive care unit when every vital system in his body was starting to fail. The *raison d'etre* of doctors in tertiary care hospitals is "train-wreck resurrection"—medical parlance for resuscitating gravely wounded patients—hence the consensus: we must do all in our power to save him despite being unable to fix his leukemia. And despite Dan's ringing declaration as we delivered him into the hands of our intensivists: *In two hours I'm going. Shit, let me home. Home.* Backed up by the immediate response from Tony—his biker-dad in teenage threads—*Fine, son, go for it.*

Two hours later Dan suffered a major seizure, and his lungs, liver and kidneys shut down for no apparent cause. Finally, we got it: we doctors were not in charge here. We halted all our resuscitation efforts, silenced the ventilator's constant noise, withdrew the tubes from his trachea, stomach, radial artery, bladder. Moe his mother murmured, *Thank you.* She spoke of her son in the past tense: *Dan was a fixer, he'd have fixed this if he could. We'll scatter his ashes on the Gulf where he hooked his first fish.*

The immediate prelude to Dan's death was horrendous; but the last moments of his life were blessedly peaceful. With his dying came healing—for Dan, for Tony and Moe, for all of us who cared for thim.

Part One

Immigrating

Culture Shock

A downtown Cleveland winter:
sidewalk snow to my knee, a slushy slipstream
on the street. Standing in the freeze line
for the bus, alien sights and sounds assail me,
the numbness skirring about my head,
inklings of terror urgently swept into the mist.

Immigrant, 2002

In mid-December 1978, my TWA jet touched down in Cleveland Hopkins international airport. I was thirty-six and had arrived from London on a one-way ticket. My new boss Sam Gross greeted me effusively and led me to the car park through a two-lane highway tunneled between ten-foot banks of snow. I'd been hired two months earlier by a buddy of Sam's, an urbane infectious disease specialist who broke his vacation to meet me on the steps of the British Museum. We had shaken on the agreement that I would start work as an associate professor at Rainbow Babies & Children's Hospital by year's end.

In early July, at the crack of dawn, I ended my marriage by leaving our house in Muswell Hill toting a single suitcase. When I arrived in my new home, I was totally unprepared for the eighteen months of emptiness, inadequacy and grief that lay ahead. After three horribly alien weeks of transition in Cleveland, I escaped to the shelter of my girlfriend Barbara's home outside Columbus.

"What's going to become of me?" I wailed.

"Oh, you'll find your way. Be a full professor some place before you know it."

The thought belied belief. Where on earth did she come up with this farfetched notion? Yet within ten years she was to be proved right. “Way will open, when you get out of your own way,” Quakers say. Barbara took me that Sunday to my first Quaker meeting for worship. Twenty-odd middle-aged and older folk were gathered in a silent circle on an assortment of armchairs and dining room chairs, with five abreast on a sagging sofa—all more or less facing the giant fireplace. I had come in out of the storm into this sturdy Victorian house—a place of sanctuary.

I scanned the shelves of Quaker books and magazines as the stillness lengthened and deepened, broken occasionally by a few brief sentences, as one or other Friend “spoke to his or her condition.” Their accents were as alien as those that beset me on the hospital wards in Cleveland, but the speakers’ calm and gentle smiles gave off a loving familiarity. I had found a welcoming home among strangers.

Over my first three weeks on my new job, I had endured a cacophony of foreign sights and sounds. Sam had run me around the whole place, making endless corridor introductions to my new colleagues, whose names and jobs I promptly forgot on our headlong dash in and out of elevators. Each morning, I struggled to follow the patient updates delivered at breakneck speed by the interns, as the weighty patient charts and X-rays found their way down the length of the table in the doctors’ lounge. Welcome to culture shock. No one had thought to warn me.

I didn’t even know what Tylenol was (Panadol in Britain), so how could I begin to interpret the endless shorthand acronyms penned by the interns into a young teenager’s chart—*13 WM c/o CP, SOB 1 wk PTA*—? I would gradually piece together the meanings of these phrases of “medicalese” from perusing countless charts, overhearing conversations among the nurses and other staff, and even having the patients explain to me what was wrong with them. My best stab at the above phrase was *“thirteen-year-old white male, complaining of chest pain, shortness of breath, for one week prior to admission.”* But I couldn’t possibly bring myself to verify this with some passing intern.

Now here I was breathing easy for the first time on American soil among these peaceful Friends in Barbara's Columbus meeting house. After the hour's silent worship, my new friends/Friends listened with no apparent judgment to my story over tea and cookies, unwittingly offering a place where I could begin to shed my cumulative grief. Grief, I was soon to realize, that I had kept deeply buried since my mother's death in my early adolescence.

It was caring for children with life-limiting—too often life-taking—illnesses that became the source of my greatest solace. Their courage and resilience, their acceptance of the hand fate had dealt them, never ceased to inspire me. Though some recovered to lead healthy lives and in time bring their own babies to meet me, many did not. It had never been in my job description to sit on their beds at the end of my working day, to hear about their lives and to share something of my own. But it was there that I came to touch the core of intimate relationship. Part of me felt a profound sense of failure at my oftentimes ineffective treatments, but faced with a child's incurable cancer, I also knew my presence served a purpose. The transition from busy fixer to silent witness, from objective professional to listening companion, held deep healing for both of us.

Bejeysus

2AM on the phone. A hard hail of
Fear hits me, icing the voice…
She asks me over: Why's he getting worse?

Fear, 2002

That first winter in Cleveland, Ohio, was the hardest transition of my life. It took two months for my car to arrive from London, so I often had to wait on the sidewalk outside Rainbow Babies and Children's Hospital for the bus to drop me off two blocks from my apartment in Shaker Heights. The snow drifts would reach to my knees as I plowed my way home after enduring another day of alien sights and voices. I was almost always the only white person on the bus, and I barely understood a word my companions were saying. After a few trips I started to recognize a few black faces, but I was too embarrassed by my BBC English accent to attempt conversation. And what could we possibly talk about? What could we possibly have in common?

My very first night on call, the phone roused me from a restless sleep at two in the morning.

"Why do they do this to a person? You bring 'em up to behave, wipe their noses, then they go and get sick and scare the mallacht outta ye."

In my dazed state I thought at first the voice must be coming straight from Killarney, County Kerry. Then I quickly recalled it: my caller was the mother of a boy who had had me jumping through hoops a few hours earlier. As she continued shouting down the phone—"Why's he getting worse? When will his fever break? Will the seizures come back?"—I felt an unexpected warmth start to fill me. Because she and her family were new immigrants, too.

I had at once felt a kind of kinship with them, amidst a cacophony of Midwestern accents, even though they hailed from Dublin, not London. I learned later that *mallacht* meant a curse. Her husband had just been posted to the local branch of the international company he worked for, only for Billy, their five-year-old, to be hit with leukemia. He had been responding well to his initial treatment until he suffered a prolonged epileptic seizure late one evening, There was no obvious explanation. We had carried out a battery of tests—a lumbar puncture to exclude meningitis, a CAT scan to make sure there was no bleeding into his brain, as well as extensive blood work. We were no nearer an explanation, so put Billy's fit down to a simple "febrile seizure"—something not uncommon in young children with high fevers, and needing no further explanation.

Sometimes the very absence of serious findings can be reassuring: better a negative result than the uncovering of raging meningitis or a hemorrhage into the brain in one so vulnerable. After reassuring myself and—I'd vainly hoped—his mother, that Billy was recovering well, and that he was getting all the necessary drugs to forestall further fits and treat every infection we could think of, I opted to head home for a couple of hours' sleep. But if I thought his mom was ready to settle down too, I was way wrong. After I'd left the unit, she had stayed wide awake and alert at his bedside, highly skeptical of my reassurances and of our negative tests. In the early hours, unable to stand the suspense any longer, she had snaffled my phone number from the nurses' station and called me up. So there I was, struggling in my groggy condition to offer a few words of comfort. Mostly I just propped myself up in bed on one elbow and silently heard her out.

"You're not certain, then? Don't ye know what's goin' on?" I could hear her frenzied voice clearly over the thundering wind and snow beyond my bedroom window. It didn't help any to recite once more that all our tests had turned out normal and we were doing all we could to pilot her son through these rocky waters. The voice remained flint hard. Unaccountably, its sound had jerked loose a long-suppressed memory of a schoolmaster from my tenth grade, who sought every pretext to stoop close to my right ear and yell fearfully into it at the barest provocation. This unwelcome recollection didn't help my already shaky professional demeanor on the end of the line.

But my silence finally achieved something I scarcely deserved. Far from deciding she was talking to a mute pudding-head who had no business caring for her sick son, she seemed to sense a calm and attentive ear. After several more minutes of this largely one-way conversation, her words started to loosen and flow more freely.

"It's workin', isn't it? Ye know, don't ye?"

Her voice was quieting with every word. I was no longer hearing that angry schoolmaster pounding down on my adolescent energy. At last, after her seemingly ceaseless tirade—while I lay back on my pillow with my eyes closed, doing my best to deflect this sweep of terror and admit a tiny hint of hopefulness—she became utterly calm.

"Glad we talked, Doc. Thanks for listening."

With these unlooked-for words of appreciation she hung up.

Indigenous wisdom reminds us that we have two eyes, two ears, two nostrils, and one mouth—and that we should use them in that proportion. Sometimes, maybe more often than not, keeping quiet is the way to go. It can help another sort themselves out and get to where they need to be. And listening, especially in the middle of the night, can be a whole lot easier than filling the air with explanations where there are none. The sad fact is that when our patients are telling their stories, it takes us doctors less than a minute to butt in—at least, that's what the research tells us.

A few days later, when the fevers and seizures were a thing of the past, I sat on the end of Billy's bed chatting with him and his mom. This was perhaps the first time I'd felt comfy sitting—quite uninvited—on a patient's bed. Mom and I had even got around to sharing a bit about our experiences as newcomers to this mighty industrial American city. All at once she reached into her carryall bag, shyly unfolded and handed me a piece of paper. It had a short poem written on it—the first poem, it turned out, that she had written since her own childhood. The scrawled lines brought me openly to tears.

Why do they do this to a person? ... the craziness of kids, scaring us both like this ... son, read the book where it says, after the bit about brushing your teeth ... the bit about not having fits—and giving us fits.

Poetry therapy at its best, it seemed to me. Given a little time to reflect, and the chance to spill out her first fears—thinly masked as anger—onto me, Billy's mother had been able to pin down her confused thoughts and feelings and make simple and elegant sense of them. Best of all, she had managed to add a strong dash of healing humour to the mix. As the emergency passed, she must have felt a need to write something about this fearful episode, to shed any lingering emotion and to make it a safer and happier memory to recall.

The crafting of a poem is a simple enough prescription for dealing with all manner of physical, emotional, and spiritual trauma. Poetry therapist John Fox calls poem-making "revelation, resurrection, and rebirth ... when we listen to each other we meet in the place of intuitive knowing." Putting a creative pen to paper is a God-given gift we all have, if we want to accept it. I too have found telling a story with the best words I can find helps me lay a lingering and bothersome memory to rest. This woman hadn't read any textbooks about writing with healing purpose; it was simply a mother's instinct that told her it would help to put these few words on paper to mark the event. As for me, my brain may not have been functioning too well that night, but my heart was with Billy's mother all the way. Maybe she sensed this, and it helped her more than any amount of brain power could have done.

The Teacher

"I haven't been around too many people with sickle cell, so maybe you can teach me some"

The pediatric residents who were making patient rounds with me soon after I arrived at Rainbow Babies & Children's introduced me to my first "sickler." *Sickler* is a pejorative though freely used shortening for someone suffering from sickle cell anaemia, which affects about eighty-thousand people in the United States alone. I had to learn fast if I was to save face in front of this band of smart and experienced resident doctors, who knew all there was to know about this disease—because I'd never cared for a single sufferer during my whole five-year pediatric fellowship in Glasgow. The reason was simple: in the 1970s, it was unusual in the West of Scotland to meet people of African descent. And during my two years working on the Barts (St. Bartholomew's) faculty right before emigrating to America, my work was confined to caring for young people with cancer.

These young US-ers were well accustomed to dealing with a lengthy roster of affected patients, because many young ones with sickle cell disease were frequent visitors to the emergency department, mostly after dark and especially when the weather turned cold. It was now late January, and we had just suffered another heavy whiteout, the third of the winter. But Dylan was perhaps not the best patient for me to learn from. I could tell as I approached his bedside that it was going to be tough to rouse him from his slumber and strike up a coherent conversation. He was hooked to an IV line containing a mix of morphine and Ativan, a potent sedative and antianxiety drug, which was being infused around the clock.

"We've tried weaning him every day since he got here," his intern told me. "As soon as he half-wakes up he starts yelling that the pain is still killing him. It took us two weeks last time he was in." He paused and looked at me as though I might have imported some new and magic bullet across the Atlantic to add to his armamentarium. "We'd sure be open to new ideas."

Putting me firmly on the spot. I was not about to admit my ignorance of even the standard approaches to sickle cell crises. I'd spent the last several minutes silently dredging up my scant knowledge from my medical school textbooks of more than ten years distance in time. I knew sickle cell anaemia was inherited, and that patients were born with a permanent defect of the hemoglobin in their red blood cells, which would get bent out of their normal healthy shape under conditions of stress. This in turn led to blocking up of the smallest blood vessels by these distorted red cells, causing prolonged and excruciating pain as one vital tissue after another became progressively starved of oxygen. It was very much like frostbite, and it was all too clear that these crises could last a good long time. At this point I had no idea for just how long.

The resident took my silence for a dearth of new notions as he led me out into the corridor. "I guess we'll just keep going then. This guy's a regular repeater. I hear things aren't great at home, and now he's out of school he's gotta find time hanging heavy. Probably likes it better in here. Pain seeker if you ask me."

I had no idea what he meant by "pain seeker," but I wasn't about to quiz him. Maybe I could find it described in some book somewhere.

"How old is he?" By the look of him he couldn't be much more that fourteen, so what did the resident mean by being "out of school"?

"Just had his nineteenth birthday."

Another piece of knowhow I would acquire when I got my hands on that hematology textbook: teenagers with sickle cell disease often don't grow well, or even have noticeable puberty spurts—though no one seems quite sure why. Just another unwelcome aspect of this horrid illness. After rounds, I found my way back to Dylan's room, hoping to begin my hands-on education about sickle cell disease with the man himself. He surely had to be pretty well informed after his nineteen years of suffering its plagues. I managed to partially rouse him after a few gentle nudges. "I know you're sleepy, Dylan, but I wanted to chat a bit. And I hear you've been sleeping solidly for a good few days. Maybe you can tell me something about what's been happening."

"Who wants to know?" His look was sulky, and he made no effort to open his eyes.

"I'm a new doctor here. I'm in charge on the ward this week."

"Shit, another new one. I just got used to those old guys. Not that they're much use to me."

"Seems like you're having a tough time, eh?"

He didn't offer up any response to this.

"So this happens a lot to you, I hear. Pain crises."

"Hey, goes with the effing territory, right? I got stuck with this effing disease, and I end up spending half my life in this dungeon. Just my crap luck. And all they do is stick me on those painkillers which half the time don't work diddly-shit …" He trailed off, hauled his sheet and blankets up over his shoulders, and closed his eyes once more.

"I'm sorry, Dylan. I wish we could do more. Seems we don't have too many answers." I ventured to pull my chair a bit closer. "But I'm going to look into things some, see what's new out there."

"Whole lot of good that's gonna do. You don't get over sickle cell, so I'm stuck with it. Pains in my feet, pains in my chest, pains in my butt, you name it."

I couldn't come up with anything else to say in the face of this pity party. I guess the resident docs were right: Dylan was a tough case in more ways than one.

"Stuck me back up in Intensive last time. My lungs were about choking. Came close to dying of pneumonia. Might have been better off if I had. Then there's a bunch of new guys down in Emerg every few months. Don't know shit about it, but they never have my chart handy. And they're for sure not about to ask the nurses anything about me. They look at all the scars on my arms, and then they can't get an IV started. So, of course I have to be some kind of drug addict, don't I? Or worse, a pusher. Doesn't help I know all my drugs real well, even the doses. So I tell them what I need, and how maybe they could give me a supply of Oxycontin to keep me out of here. That really gets 'em going."

He trailed off, grabbed a box of tissues from the bed table, and started trying to hawk up tacky spit. He grasped his ribs and winced with the pain that the coughing was bringing on. I sat back, wondering how I could begin to deal with all this anger, this resentment at the world—at even being born, it seemed like.

The door swung open and a young nurse appeared. A stunner, with skin the colour of dark roasted coffee. "Hi, Dylan. I'm your new nurse this evening. Hanna." She stopped. "Sorry, Doctor, I didn't know you were here. I can come back."

"No, no. It's fine. We were just chatting."

But Dylan had lost all interest in chatting with me—if he ever had any. He clearly couldn't keep his eyes off the newcomer.

"Just got to check your vitals. How's the pain, Dylan? Mind if I call you Dylan?"

His expression had changed to one of rank astonishment, as if anyone would ever ask his permission about anything.

"Sure," he mumbled. "Not so good. Well, I guess it's eased some."

He hadn't been about to acknowledge that to me. Maybe a little male pride was kicking in. Hanna moved to the other side of the bed to check the IV settings, then ventured to perch on the edge of his bed to check his temp and pulse rate.

"Everything's looking good from our viewpoint, Dylan. Is there anything I can do for you? I haven't been around too many people with sickle cell, so maybe you can teach me some."

Why couldn't I have come right out and said that? But I guess it's a whole lot easier when you're a young nurse starting out than when you're the guy who's supposed to be in charge and calling the shots. Dylan's surly look had utterly vanished, replaced by an almost childlike softness. The young nurse's kindness had clearly got to him—that and her gorgeous looks, no doubt. I eased back in my chair and let their conversation unfold.

"Yeah, sure. I know about everything there is to know. It's a killer, I'll tell you that."

"D'you get many people come see you, Dylan?"

"What's it look like? My mom, she's probably out with her latest. And my dad, he's been gone forever—we're not in touch. I can't hardly keep in touch with my buds, what with being in and out of this place."

"No girlfriends?"

"I never had a date," he whispered. "No girl's ever going to want me."

"Don't you be so sure. Lots of girls want to hang out with guys who've had more than their share of tough breaks."

"Life sucks, you know it?" Now Dylan looked on the point of tears.

Hanna stayed quiet, then laid a hand on his arm. "I'm real sorry this happened to you. I hear you're in here quite a bit. I expect I'll be looking after you again."

"That'd be good."

"Listen, there's something I don't usually share with my patients," the nurse went on. "My last year in high school, I got this bad gut problem. Ulcerative colitis they call it. Often comes on about that age. Make a long story short, I had to have this massive surgery, ended up with a stoma, around my nineteenth birthday. Some birthday gift."

To both Dylan's and my astonishment, she promptly stood up, pulled up her smock and eased down the rim of her pants. Underneath, there was a long pink scar, and a colostomy pouch was lying snug against the right side of her abdomen.

"That's what they call a stoma. It's where the poop goes. I get to empty it several times a day. The surgeons thought they could maybe hook me back up together again, but it turned out the surgery would be too dodgy, so I'm stuck with it. Like forever." She tugged up her pants, dropped her smock back in place, and grinned at both of us. "But what I want to tell you, Dylan, it hasn't screwed up my social life one bit. One guy got turned off when he found out, but that relationship wasn't going anywhere anyway."

Dylan was struck dumb, his face lit with admiration.

"Guess you never know what life's going to hand you," Hanna finished up. "Just have to deal with it. But I know you can do that, Dylan. I'm rooting for you."

I found myself grinning for no apparent reason throughout the rest of my morning rounds. Even if I wasn't going to learn much from the resident doctors, how lovely to discover what a caring and fun teaching resource the Rainbow nurses could be. And I'd just witnessed healing in the form of a pretty face and loving words.

Then I met Charlene. She had been diagnosed with sickle cell disease as an infant and had been making frequent trips into Rainbow ever since. I met her for the first time when she was eight, and this had been an especially tough winter for her. She had had five separate admissions, each of them triggered by an infection and each lasting many days. She would spike high temperatures, usually accompanied by a wracking cough that kept her from a peaceful night's sleep—and all too often, from getting enough oxygen to fuel her frail little body.

The most recent episode was the worst. School was about to get out for Christmas when she came home holding her ribs and her belly. Sometimes her mother was able to ease things with a glass of warm milk and a heating pad over whatever part of her body was hurting. She gave Charlene a couple of Tylenol with codeine pills and had her lie down on the sofa in front of the TV while she warmed a drink for her. In the time-honoured way of mothers the world over, she tried humming Charlene's favorite song while gently rubbing her belly and her back to see if she could make things better. As was her wont, Charlene offered not a word of complaint and struggled to muster a smile. But when her mother checked her temperature this time and saw it was reading 102°, she knew there was only one solution: call the hospital.

Just as her schoolmates were gearing up for last-minute Christmas preparations, Charlene was once more on her way into Rainbow. By the time they reached our Emergency Room, Charlene's pains had moved up to her chest and she was having trouble breathing freely. The resident called me after he had checked her out.

"Her oxygen's reading ninety-one on the monitor. Suggests a big problem with getting enough air into her lungs. We've got her hooked up to the supplemental oxygen supply on the wall, and I just called the radiology tech in to X-ray her chest."

The chest X-ray showed that much of the little girl's healthy lungs had been replaced by gathering white clouds that made it hard to distinguish the outlines of her heart. She was showing all the signs of what is known as an acute chest syndrome, meaning that the small blood vessels of her lungs were becoming choked with sickle cells. This in turn allowed bacteria to move swiftly in and set up pneumonia in the areas where the blood had ceased to flow. Where there is poor blood flow there is poor defense against infection.

The standard treatment for this condition is with exchange blood transfusion. The idea is to wash out as much of the patient's blood as possible, taking with it most of the sickle cells blocking up the little blood vessels, while replacing them temporarily with healthy donor red blood cells that will hang around long enough to see them through the immediate crisis. These children also need potent antibiotics, because less frequent infections like mycoplasma can sometimes be the culprit. They also need extra oxygen by face mask, or even through artificial ventilation if this is not enough to raise their blood oxygen to a safe level. Any worries that morphine and similar drugs may suppress breathing efforts must never hold us back from giving big enough doses to ease the severe chest pain these patients suffer.

Exchange transfusion, plus a lot of intravenous antibiotics, extra oxygen, and enough pain medication, are usually enough for children suffering from an acute chest syndrome to pull through it. But it's always touch and go. I met with Charlene's mother and grandma in the ER for the first time. Children with severe illnesses get very sick very quick, and as an oncologist one thing I've had a lot of practice at is meeting parents for the first time whose children show up close to death. I explained the urgency of the situation as gently but as urgently as I could, and exactly what we had to do if Charlene was to make it. The little girl was adjusting to her tight-fitting oxygen mask and her breathing had slowed a little. She was trying to ask me something, but her voice was muffled by the mask. I leaned in close to her face.

"Can I keep my dolly here?" For the first time I noticed what she had tucked up under her arm: a rag doll complete with kerchief and red and white striped apron. It bore a striking resemblance to Charlene's grandma.

"You bet you can. She'll look after you if you get scared. What's her name?"

"Matilda," she whispered back. And after a pause: "Thank you."

Where did this eight-year-old girl, who must be terrified and in great pain, find it in herself to thank me for such a tiny gift? She had to have been born with an attitude of gratitude.

We transported Charlene directly from the ER to the pediatric intensive care unit where the exchange transfusion would take place. An extremely difficult and scary procedure for an eight-year-old, especially because it meant putting not just one but two catheters into her fragile veins. This was essential to allow the exchange transfusion to extract and replace a high enough percentage of the sickled red blood cells. If we'd wondered how Charlene would handle the whole procedure, we had reckoned without this young girl's fortitude, and that of her family.

Once they had made it to the ICU, her mother clasped one of her daughter's hands tight and I held onto the other. By God's grace the resident managed after a lot of poking and prodding to insert the catheters and get blood flowing freely through each. There was never a squirm or a whimper from Charlene throughout. She continued breathing as slowly and deeply as she could through her mask, only the tightening of her grip around my fingers betraying her anguish. Matilda was tucked firmly under one arm, her head peeking out over the bedclothes. The steady rhythm of the blood exchange machine finally lulled Charlene to a fitful slumber.

By the next morning, her breathing was significantly easier, but I could tell her sides and back were still hurting. I perched gingerly on the edge of her bed, knowing the pressure of the blankets could only add to her pain.

"How're you doing, Charlene?"

"Better today," she whispered.

"Did you manage to eat anything?"

"Yeah, they gave me some cereal. Fruit loops." It seemed important to let me know specifics about the content of her breakfast.

"That's good. Did they give you enough medicine for your pain?"

"Mm-hm. Thanks."

No way was she ever going to complain. I couldn't help remembering Dylan and his bitter attitude toward his illness. Hard to know which came first in Charlene—this attitude of gratitude that seemed inborn in her, or her learned response to her family's constant love. Her dad's parents lived out of state, but as soon as they heard their granddaughter was so ill, they had driven through the night to be there with her. The family members took turns to be at her bedside.

The next morning, Charlene was well enough to be moved back down to our pediatric ward. When I checked on her late in the day, my friend and colleague, Jill Sonke, and one of her students, were with her. Jill is our dancer-in-residence at the hospital, and as a teenager with a serious illness herself she had known what it was like to suffer a painful and debilitating illness that kept you in bed for long periods. She had brought her scarves along—numerous brightly coloured diaphanous sheets of silk that she uses to create dances that a bed-bound child could take part in. Charlene was holding onto the end of one of the larger scarves, waving it up and down in time as Jill's student beat out the rhythm on a conga drum, and Jill swept gracefully under and over the scarf. Charlene would giggle, then wince when the pain caught her. But I knew better than to suggest upping the morphine and putting her out of it: her delight in this communal dancing was at least as therapeutic as any more opioid therapy.

Later that day, her mother brought Charlene's two brothers in to see her. They had just got out of school for the Christmas vacation and were bubbling over with all that was going on at home. Their daddy had brought a tree home that day, and they had pulled out the big box of decorations from its safe place in their utility room cupboard.

"We're going to wait till you get home, though, Char," her younger brother, Michael, assured her.

"You don't have to," she said. "I don't know when I'm coming home."

She looked wistfully at her mom, but she didn't say anything else. There were only three days to go until Christmas, and Charlene was receiving a further transfusion and was still hooked up to her IV antibiotics. Although she had come through the worst, I wasn't at all sure she would make it out for the 25th. Her grandparents and mother alternated spending time at her bedside, and her dad would bring the boys in each afternoon after he had finished work. Everyone on the staff enjoyed spending a few extra minutes in Charlene's room.

Her graceful acceptance of all that was happening to her inspired everyone, and there were always games and other activities going on around her. Gradually she could get up to the bathroom and eat a little soup and pudding, and we were able to give her antibiotics and pain meds by mouth. I visited her late in the afternoon on Christmas Eve.

"Charlene, I think we might be able to send you home tomorrow morning."

She still looked weak and frail, but there was no mistaking her grin.

"Well, if you can't make it out tomorrow, we'll just bring Christmas to you right here," her mother added.

The charge nurse greeted me when I got in the next morning. "Charlene had her first good night's sleep since she's been here. Are you going to let her home for Christmas?"

"Sounds like it to me." When I poked my head around the door, I saw Charlene already had her street clothes on.

“Looks like you made the decision already, hon. You think you’re ready to go?”

She nodded her head emphatically.

“I think she’s ready, Doctor,” her mother said. “She slept almost the whole night through. And she ate some grits and drank some juice this morning already.”

We all gathered to see Charlene off that Christmas morning. She shook hands with each of the resident doctors and nurses who had looked after her, thanking each one in turn. She had a small present for each, with her handwriting on the wrapping paper. But watching her daddy push her wheelchair into the elevator was Christmas enough for all of us.

A Late Arrival

"Don't make a habit of importing sick patients from South America"

A few minutes after five o'clock on a Friday evening in the pediatric hematology oncology office. Our secretaries had vanished with their customary promptness, and I was about to follow them when the phone on Maureen's desk rang. I knew the voice machine would be turned on and as the on-call doctor I would get the message soon enough if I was needed. But I picked it up anyway. It was the Delta check-in desk at Gainesville airport.

"Sir, we're looking for one of the doctors," an official voice said. "I think a hematologist. One for children."

I took in the phrases as they unfolded. He had hit the exact right button on the keyboard. I wondered briefly how many times he had been shuffled around by our switchboard operators.

"That's me."

"Well, we have a young lady here with her baby. She says the baby has leukemia."

Usually when a new patient comes to us there is at least a preliminary call from the referring doctor. I had had no such message.

"Did she say where she'd come from?"

"Guyana. It's in South America somewhere."

I knew exactly where it was. I'd been a stamp collector since I was six years old, and collected stamps from every British colony, dating from before each one of them had declared their independence. Guyana was once British Guiana but had gained its freedom from British rule in 1966, the same year that I graduated from medical school. That meant the mother would speak English, because Guyana is the only South American country where English is still the official language.

"How does the baby look to you?" I quizzed the Delta guy.

"Well, sir, she's asleep in her crib right now, but she seems okay."

"Has the mom got enough money for a cab?"

"Yeah, I checked on that. She's got a couple of hundred dollars. And her passport is in order."

"Did she say how she knows her baby has leukemia?"

"She said she saw the doctors in her hometown when the baby took sick, and they gave her medicine for what they said was leukemia. But it seems it stopped working. The mom doesn't look too well herself," he added.

I covered the phone and allowed myself an audible sigh. This sounded like a mess. A child with a very uncertain diagnosis from a developing country, presumably with no other family here, reaching out for help. How the mother had found us I couldn't imagine. I let myself wonder how many other such children were out there in countries where the medical services were limited to comfort care at best. Then felt instantly ashamed of my thought—I knew only too well what it felt like to be an immigrant in a strange country. But I had had a much sought-after job waiting for me. And I certainly hadn't had the responsibility for a young daughter with what sounded like a life-threatening illness. Kate and George were safe and sound with their mom back in London.

"You think it's safe for them to travel by cab—rather than send an ambulance for them?"

"Yes, I think so."

He sounded like he was used to dealing with the unexpected—even emergencies. I made a quick decision.

“Can you put them in a cab and direct it over to Shands Emergency Room? We’ll be looking for them. What’s the name?” I added as an afterthought.

“Benitez. The child’s name is Angelina. She’s a beautiful little thing. Do your best, Doc.”

Delta had not been overstating it about Angelina’s mom not looking too well. When I first saw the two of them tucked together in a chair in the corner of one of the ER rooms, my first impression was of a pale rake-thin woman, consumed by racking coughs every few minutes. She was doing the best she could to shield them from the child sleeping restlessly in her arms. How long had this sick woman been caring singlehanded for her gravely sick child?

“Her temp’s thirty-nine-point-five,” her nurse told me. “BP’s a bit marginal too.”

I wondered briefly whose vitals the nurse was reporting on—child or mom?

“Want me to call PICU?”

“Yeah. Let’s get some fluids started, blood work—CBC, blood culture, lytes, LFT’s. She needs a chest film too.” I turned to the pediatric resident who had just joined us. “Can you get your opposite number in Internal Medicine in here once you’ve gone over Angelina? We need to get Mom some help too.”

Between shaking coughs, Angelina’s mother quizzed me in her singsong accent.

“Doctor, can you help her? They told me they couldn’t do any more for her. They gave her medicine, but it stopped working.”

“We’re going to do all we can, Mrs. Benitez. But first we need to find out more about Angelina. Do you have any papers with you from the doctors who took care of her?”

Angelina remained on the edge between life and death for three days. Her blood cultures confirmed septicemia, and her blood count and bone marrow showed leukemia raging out of control. Meanwhile her mother had been admitted to an isolation room two floors below: her chest X-ray had shown active TB. Mercifully—almost unbelievably—there was no sign that she had infected her daughter. As the radiologist and I gazed at Angelina's healthy lungs on the X-ray screen, I offered up thanks for this small blessing.

But we had to start right in with our chemo if there was to be any chance for Angelina. A calculated risk because of the damage on any normal blood cells the chemo would immediately trigger. But like so many desperately ill young ones, Angelina defied the odds. Impossible to imagine what was going on inside the head of this fifteen-month-old, surrounded by strangers in an alien world, torn from the arms of her mother, hooked up to all the paraphernalia of 21st-century high-tech medicine. But a week after she had arrived at Gainesville airport, sick almost to death and accompanied by her very sick mom, I came into Angelina's room to find her sitting up and playing with Emma, one of our child life specialists, along with a big woolly white bear.

She didn't want anything to do with me, and at once started to cry when I perched on the end of her bed. Not such a bad sign—a normal enough reaction of a toddler to a strange doctor. The scars from needle sticks on her frail arms spoke to the trauma of the last few weeks. I got off the bed and knelt down beside it instead—hopefully a less frightening pose. A few more prayers on my part wouldn't come amiss either.

"Looks like you two are making friends," I said to Emma.

"She's pretty shell-shocked by all that's been happening, John. And she cries for her mom a lot. Don't you, hon?" Emma kept her voice light and her eyes on Angelina, still playing with the toy bear that was big enough to almost conceal the little girl in the bed.

A week later, after talking to the internists we decided her mother was responding well enough to her anti-TB drugs that the benefit of reuniting her with her daughter outweighed any risk of spreading her infection. Angelina meanwhile was responding to our treatment and was out of any immediate danger. Mom and daughter were cuddled up in bed together, both wearing masks, when I made my morning rounds. Emma was sitting on the other side of the bed.

"We've been talking about some things," she told me. "I hear Angelina could be ready to leave the hospital soon. Maybe we can all talk about what comes next?"

We had started to discuss this over the past few days. Gloria, Angelina's mother, was terrified of the idea of returning home, and I knew she was right. Judging by the state that both of them were in when they first touched down in Gainesville airport, neither could get the kind of care they needed back in Guyana. Angelina needed further intensive treatment over at least the next six months to stand the remotest chance of ridding her of her leukemia for good. Even then the odds were far from great. She had received woefully inadequate initial treatment and had swiftly relapsed. We had found leukemia cells in her spinal fluid as well as her bone marrow, a not uncommon complication but one that added to the complexity of her therapy.

"They can stay in Rush Lake for a few weeks at least," Emma said, referring to a nearby motel we sometimes used for patients who couldn't safely be housed in our Ronald McDonald House. "Gloria has some money, and her husband is sending more."

We all knew this wasn't a long term answer. The family had less than two months left on their visa. What we needed was legal advice. I had had a few conversations with an immigration lawyer in town about my own status. Though by then I had lived in the United States for several years, I still held the green card of a resident alien. I had met Jill, a very savvy immigration lawyer, at a Christmas party and started the conversation about what kind of documentation I would need. I called her the following morning.

"The biggest thing will be a strong letter from you," she told me. "I have dozens of cases lined up, and the INS is getting pickier and pickier. We can try plucking at their heartstrings, and stress how much the State of Florida has already invested in this family. Their papers are all in order, you say?"

"Yup. They're good people. Dad is an accountant back home, and I understand Mom was working fulltime until the baby got sick. They have quite a bit of money."

"How did they end up in Gainesville?"

"It turns out Mom put "Florida" and "University" together and came up with us. It happens every so often."

In the end, it took a series of letters, and laborious negotiations between Jill and the INS, but close to a year later the family had gained resident alien status and had got themselves housed in a small apartment. Gloria was cleared of infection and had found a job at a local garden nursery. I made a habit of dropping by on my way home. It was quickly evident that Gloria was fitting in well in her new surroundings. The most gratifying thing of all was that Angelina continued to respond to our treatments and had become to all intents and purposes a healthy toddler. As to the medical and hospital bills, I had somehow persuaded our hospital administrators to write off almost everything, bar a nominal sum that the family was able to pay off in small installments.

"But don't make a habit of importing any more desperately sick patients from South America," the VP for budgets remonstrated.

I reflected that I hadn't exactly gone out and touted for the Benitez family's business, but kept the thought to myself.

Part Two

Learning from the Young

Midder

"the origin of our human race—as sacred a mystery as the moment of death"

My love for children was born on my *midder* rotation: English med school slang for midwifery. In March 1964, I was dispatched to the North Middlesex Hospital in Enfield, North London, accompanied by my equally wet-behind-the-ears medical student colleague, Cedric, to learn the rudiments of childbirth. It's only two generations ago that Britain's midwives were still our primary mentors in the art of birthing babies.

The word *midwife* goes back at least to 1300 AD, meaning "a woman who stands with" a birthing woman and her baby, and in the West the profession of midwifery dates back to Ancient Egypt and Classical Greece. For millennia, women sat supported by birthing chairs to birth their babies through the natural impulse of gravity. British midwives mostly worked in outlying community hospitals and dedicated childbirth centres because that was where most mothers had their babies. Nowadays, the whole thing has been largely taken over by doctors, who call it obstetrics, a word adopted only in nineteenth-century Britain from the modern Latin word for the science of midwifery. Though Aristotle admired midwives for their wisdom and dedication, today their role is dominated by hospital-based obstetricians who tend to see pregnancy as a pathological condition. How did we men get in on this quintessentially female act—once we had played out our minor though necessary part in a baby's creation?

My month at the North Middlesex was a time of rapture. A callow twenty-two-year-old, I would often found myself the sole attendant at a delivery, my *accouchement* stool giving me a front-row seat as newborns slipped and slid their way into our world, with little prompting from me. For our first couple of days,

Dave Shand, the world-weary senior house officer, casually tossed me and Cedric odd crumbs of obstetrical lore, while hefting yet another pregnant lady's legs up into the stirrups for the endless series of pelvic exams somehow considered vital to modern antenatal care. But by the third day, he was leaving us to the tender care of the motherly midwives.

Even more astounding, on the principle of "see one, do one, teach one," these midwives were soon leaving me to *stand with* the birthing mom. Perhaps this was because most of our learning took place between noon on Fridays and six on Saturday mornings—the time the babies mostly chose to alight on earth. Maybe they liked the idea of starting out life on a weekend? In those days they were left largely in charge to tick by their own biological clocks, and they seemed in no hurry to leave the blissful comfort of their watery wombs. Today's obstetricians would respond to such tardiness by infusing the mom-to-be with Pitocin to speed up her contractions, if not whisking her straight off to the operating room for a Caesarian section. The babies would let everyone in listening distance know only too well what they thought of this rough treatment. Is it any surprise that their universal greeting to the world is to scream loud and long? Indeed, the absence of such fury would cause consternation all around.

Friday evenings, when most of my med student buddies would be hitting the pubs, often found me perched between the legs of a multiparous mom on a low accouchement or birthing stool. I was placed "in the breach" and the stool's casters would swivel freely on their own axis. This raised the distinct possibility of my pivoting backwards or—much worse—forwards. The midwives showed up less and less often to check on me—as much because of the "nothing-to-it" multiparity of our charges as any great faith in my skills. It was quite customary for Mom-to-be's mom or sister to be entertaining three or four toddlers in the waiting room. Even more astounding, these seasoned women themselves seemed to utterly trust me in my crucial role. As the product of a boys-only boarding school, I was unversed in the ways of the world, and it took me a dizzying few days to recover from my first full-frontal views of female anatomy in its gravid state.

Even under my mask, anyone could tell I was of very tender years to be placed in a position of such responsibility. If I had grown up in the United States I would have been carded until I was thirty. So I loved that few women ever questioned my credentials, or showed embarrassment at baring their bodies before me. Another striking difference from the US, where even senior doctors are quizzed on their every decision—though this trend towards skepticism among our public has perhaps become rife in Britain too.

But faced with such awesome responsibilities for bringing forth new life, I quickly left behind my adolescent self-doubt and found myself taking charge. I delivered three babies in one twenty-four-hour spell, snatching brief in-between naps on the couch in the nurses' lounge. I was on a lasting high—a mix of pride in my newfound skills and joy amounting almost to ecstasy as I became a servant in this mysterious act of birth. I didn't think of it then, but I now see this God-given ritual—the very origin of our human race—as a sacred mystery as momentous as the moment of our death.

Once I had the thing down, I eased into the role essentially of witness, and learned to intervene only enough to guide the baby's progress as and when needed. I spent more time getting to know these awesome women, doing all I could to relieve their physical pain, so that they too could capture some of the joy of it. Most of the mothers, it's true, were either too exhausted or too used to these delivery room encounters to have much resource for enjoyment. But even those who had been through this laborious business up to a dozen times responded to the moment of delivery with deep pride at their accomplishment and breathless delight at uniting with their new offspring.

For me, too, the crowning point was my all too brief acquaintance with these sacred new beings. How apt that the moment the head appears at the vulval entrance to announce the baby's arrival is called the crowning. With the cutting of the cord, and with their first strident cry out into the world, these slippery, bloody creatures, faces temporarily squished and scalps misshapen from their arduous trip down the birth canal, proclaimed their arrival. Their first protests behind them, they were *here*, and they were *now*. As yet untouched by the cumulative distresses of the world, they were totally free of any judgment, remorse, or despair. And I was in awe of every one of them. They seemed to have come into my life to teach me over and over again how to live. That this moment is *it*, nothing else counts. These newborns were the centre of the world's attention, as they utterly expected to be. They were bent on *love*—both on receiving their just due and on giving it right back as unconditional bounty. No wonder many mothers feel so serene when they have babies floating inside them.

But by no means every birth is a joyful experience. It can be an immense and heart-wrenching problem to judge if a newborn babe is meant to be with us here in our world. I got a call one night from the duty midwife to come urgently to the Labour & Delivery suite.

"The ambulance just brought this young girl in. She started bleeding early this evening and it looks like she's about to deliver. She claims she didn't know she was pregnant, but she must be well on judging by the looks of things. There's no family with her."

When I made it to the unit, the midwife was completing a pelvic exam on Mom. She looked about fourteen, and terrified.

"I estimate she's around thirty weeks," the midwife told me quietly. "No antenatal care at all. Babe's alive, but in a lot of distress. Heartbeat around two hundred, and very weak. It'll be touch and go."

Ten minutes later, the mother pushed her son out with scarcely a whimper. He was dusky blue and looked lifeless—about two pounds, if that. The midwife passed him into my waiting arms. Mom had subsided back into exhausted sleep, so she didn't have to watch what was going on. I rushed the small bundle of limpness over to the exam table, listened for a heartbeat as the midwife struggled to fasten an oxygen mask over his tiny face. The heartbeat was thready and too rapid for me to count. I suctioned the little mite as gently as I could, and he responded with the feeblest of cries. He took a couple of weak gasps, but with no lessening of his duskiness.

I lifted the mask an inch to offer him my finger, but he had no strength, or instinct, to suck. He needed an immediate intravenous infusion of fluids if we were going to resuscitate him, but I couldn't imagine getting a needle into those almost non-existent veins. It felt like an exercise in total futility, but we couldn't just let him die. Could we?

The midwife interrupted my pondering. "Let's get him weighed."

We unswaddled him briefly from his warm wrappings and laid him on the infant scales.

"Two pounds, four ounces," she read off. "Can't remember having one this size who made it. You'd better phone Dave Shand."

Her soft tones were suddenly comforting. I glanced up at her.

"You're right. Thanks."

Dave woke swiftly to his phone. "I'll be there in ten minutes."

I went through the motions of searching for a vein in the baby's arms, then his scalp, while I waited for Dave and the nurse prepared the IV. I made a stab with a 25-gauge needle—the smallest on offer—at what looked like a vein in the back on one hand. There was no backflow of blood, and the tissue swelling around my needle when I injected a small amount of saline told the bleak story of my futile attempt at a venipuncture. He was gasping every ten or fifteen seconds and the oxygen was maintaining a marginal pinkness, but he hadn't cried again. I felt a rush of relief when Dave appeared, examined the baby briefly, and glanced over the chart that the midwife had started.

"One-minute Apgar?"

Ah, Apgar—Virginia Apgar's score for a newborn's condition at birth. I'd completely forgotten to record it. I ran through the elements of the score swiftly in my mind—*Activity, Pulse, Grimace, Appearance, Respiration*—scoring *zero*, *one*, or *two* for each.

"One. Maybe two. He had a heartbeat, and he gasped. That's about it. No reflexes, completely floppy. Pretty much the same at five minutes."

"Pretty bad. How old's Mom?"

"Haven't been able to establish it, but she looks about fourteen."

"No Dad around? Family?"

"Nope."

"What do you think, John?"

I wasn't used to being asked my opinion on anything, though I knew Dave wasn't about to leave me to decide if this babe lived or died. Maybe he was just teaching me to think for myself?

"I think the outlook's pretty bad. Long term, I mean. Even if he survives."

"Because of the Apgar?"

"Yes. And, well, he's only about thirty weeks, could be less."

I glanced back down at the baby, who was still making rare and ineffectual gasps. I was well aware that with every minute that passed we were making the decision for him. Maybe that was Dave's intention: to play God with this fragile human life.

"The Apgar doesn't tell us too much about what might happen in his future," he commented, "whatever the books may tell you."

As he moved to reexamine the tiny form, the infant's efforts to breathe ceased altogether. Dave paused a long moment, then placed his stethoscope lightly over his chest. The baby's face and limbs were taking on a deeply cyanotic hue.

"Looks like he's made his own decision." He turned to where Mom was stirring on the bed, then scooped the baby up to lay it gently in her arms. "What's your name, dear?"

She opened her eyes, instinctively clasped her tiny newborn. "Elsie."

"Elsie, I'm very sorry, but your baby didn't make it. He just wasn't ready for this world."

A single tear rolled down Elsie's cheek. The midwife moved to her side and grasped her free hand.

"You're going to be all right. We'll keep you here a few days, till you're good and strong again, love. Can we phone your mum?"

A look of alarm spread across Elsie's face. "She doesn't know. Not even about Jimmy."

"I think she has to know. You need her right now. Is Jimmy the dad?"

"Yeah. There hasn't been nobody else." Her face crumpled and she started to sob. Dave placed a hand on Elsie's shoulder, then on the tiny form still wrapped in her arms. He glanced over at me and spoke quietly.

"You can put her in the pediatric ward, John. Check and see if the private room is empty."

Allies

She asked your pardon, voice between laughter and whimper:
"Sorry I kept you up all night."

When you look after people who come to you in life-and-death situations, you are bound to build close relationships. Not friendships exactly—more like bonds of intimacy, of shared endeavour, where there is no room for dissembling or pretense. These relationships may be as rewarding as they are essential, for the giver as much as for the receiver of care. Bonds like these can take a long time to build, and they are certainly not the norm. I suppose it's because of shyness on the part of our patients, along with all those lessons we doctors have learned so well about keeping our "professional distance." This is the psychic space we feel obligated to maintain between us and our patients.

Whatever that phrase means—I certainly wasn't given a definition in my medical school education. It is rarely encouraged by medical schoolteachers for physicians to set aside professional time even to talk—better, listen—to our patients, or even among ourselves, about the things that touch us most deeply. There is this deep-seated idea that getting too close will hamper our clinical judgment. But after all, this isn't friendship or affection we are trying to build. It's that elusive but critical thing, the doctor-patient relationship—a mix of altruism and critical objectivity. Sir William Osler called it equanimity, which you could translate as a state of "balanced mind."

Once in a while, though, the barriers drop away and doctor and patient meet soul-to-soul. That was how it was with a doctor named Anne and a patient called Shelley. After her pediatric residency in Virginia, Anne enrolled in our three-year fellowship at the University of Florida to train as a pediatric hematologist-oncologist. She combined super-competence with breathtaking Italian style and flair, while always showing deep care for her patients. I had reason to experience these qualities up close and personal one Thanksgiving weekend.

I was the attending on call with Anne in our bone marrow transplant unit. Two weeks earlier, Shelley, a fifteen-year-old patient of ours, had received a transplant to try to cure her of her leukemia. After her ultra-high doses of chemotherapy, Shelley's defenses hit rock bottom. She developed a deep muscle infection high in her right thigh, the site of an earlier catheter placement in her femoral vein, and deadly bacteria found themselves an ideal home to nest in. Though we had a bunch of antibiotics our laboratory tests told us would take care of things, these microbes clearly hadn't read the lab reports and didn't know they were supposed to crawl off and die.

An ulcer developed in Shelley's old catheter site, which tracked up into her abdomen and onwards into her anal and labial folds. Lacking a single white blood cell with which to defend herself, Shelley could make no pus—the essential sign of an effective local response to infection. The skin over the whole area turned blotchy purple, and within forty-eight hours her thigh and groin had swelled to twice their normal size. There was not a splash of healthy yellow—clear evidence that this potent cocktail of modern antibiotics was totally failing to hold the infection in check.

I knew there was already a strong bond between my young colleague and this woman on the threshold of adult life. As we discussed our options on rounds with the nurses, Anne's emotions were on the edge. After rounds were done, I pulled her aside.

"D'you think you can keep your cool enough to make objective decisions, Anne? Shelley's like your kid sister, and I have a strong hunch she's not going to make it. It can get really hard when you're that close to a patient you're caring for."

Objective means in medical parlance basing everything on proven *facts*, free of any bias or personal feelings—an odd and far from ideal word to use in these situations. But we doctors put great store in it while we are serving the mortally sick. Anne quickly set me straight.

"I'll be fine just as long as I can have a good bawl whenever I need to. Helps me keep my head on straight." She promptly burst into tears, and after a minute or two began laughing at herself. "I've always been a cry-baby. Don't mind me!"

Becky, a longtime nurse and friend to us both, had been listening in. She pushed a box of Kleenex towards Anne, while I pulled my two-foot by two-foot-square silk Union Jack handkerchief from my pants pocket—a prop I carry with me for occasions just like this. I handed it in several folds to Anne, which got the three of us laughing some more, though it was impossible to know exactly what we were guffawing about. How dare we laugh with our poor young patient suffering such pain and misery, and with all these feelings of helplessness welling up inside us? It reminded me of being overcome with a fit of the giggles at my favorite aunt's funeral service. Someone very kind said to me afterwards that I didn't have to be ashamed. It happened a lot at times like this. Tears and laughter are close neighbors—it's just that one is sometimes more *correct* than the other.

"Ah, that's better," Anne said, drying her eyes. "Now then, where were we?"

Shelley died at ten past seven the following morning; Anne had spent the night at her bedside. At one o'clock I had phoned in and offered to relieve her, but she had very matter-of-factly declined my offer.

"I've got a handle on things, John. I'm titrating up her morphine, watching I don't put her out cold. She wants to stay awake if she can." She went on to update me on every tiny medical detail—the inexorable progress of the infection, the state of her patient's kidneys and liver and lungs and brain—in as objective a way as any hardnosed medical scientist. Then: "We've been talking about her horses. And Christie's here now" (referring to Shelley's twelve year old sister). "I'm getting to know her too."

I had a brief image of the four of them—Anne, Christie, and the girls' parents—gathering in homage around their dying loved one's bed. I came on in when I got the call at seven. By the time I arrived on the unit the family was sharing their private vigil over Shelley's body. Anne was in the conference room with the two volumes of Shelley's chart. She was writing a full medical report of the events of the last twelve hours.

"I got a bit behind. Things were pretty crazy in there."

She proceeded to summarize the medical events preceding her patient's death, missing no detail of the sequence of happenings since we'd made ward rounds together the prior evening. She itemized each new crisis one-by-one and how she had handled it. Nothing was missing—she had done exactly what was needed, with both decision and compassion: a shining example of Osler's equanimity. Whatever the state of her feelings after this horrendously demanding night, she stayed every inch the consummate doctor.

"So how are *you* doing?" I asked her at last.

At once the tears welled up. "Christ, where are those Kleenex when you need them?" Then: "We talked all night. Kind of like a slumber party. She wasn't making too much sense towards the end—but she wasn't hurting any. Did you know she bred those horses herself? She and Christie. Told me all about it."

Anne kept in close touch with sister Christie and her mother, who worked in the same bank she used. A month later, she went out to visit the horses on the family's five acres north of town. She admitted to Christie that she was really scared of horses.

Which made me think: "Not much frightens you, kid. For sure not dying humans, anyway."

A Chip off the Old Block?

"Yeah, you got half your dad's genes.
But you're not your dad."

"Devon!"

The young man in the bed turned his head, tugged twitchily on the straps that had been restraining him while he was out cold.

"It's Adam. Your nurse. You hurting?"

Devon was rolling about like he was in pain, but it may have just been frustration now that he was waking up. He summoned a croak but neither Adam nor I could make out the words.

"Okay to give him more water?"

"Sure."

Adam still deferred to me—nurse-to-doctor—even though we were drinking buddies in our non-working hours. Devon licked at the drops of water on his lips when Adam squirted the bottle into his mouth.

"You're in the hospital—but you're gonna be fine, fella."

Devon opened his eyes, rolling them back and forth in search of the voice's source.

"Hard to focus, right? It's the meds, buddy. We had to calm you down—you were putting up a good fight."

"Whass … throat?"

Devon's first words came out barely articulate around the nasogastric tube.

"It's a tube, to keep your stomach empty," Adam told him. "You've been losing blood. I just gave you pain meds—they'll kick in fast."

Devon had arrived in our ER two nights earlier, after a university classmate had found him stretched out on the floor of the men's room in a pool of blood. He had been barely rousable and running a fever of 102°. We quickly identified the cause: a cancerous growth which the CAT scan had shown was almost encasing his small bowel. Almost certainly lymphoma, but our resuscitative measures had to take precedence over our pediatric surgeons getting a biopsy to confirm our suspicions.

"Time to change those sheets, Devon," Adam said. Then to me, "Give me a hand rolling him, John."

This wouldn't be the first time the two of us had made up a bed together. It was Adam who had taught me to make a perfect hospital corner. It came easy as apple pie nowadays.

"Glasses? Can't see shit."

The words were coming out much more clearly. Devon was bouncing back fast from the sedative and pain meds we had given him. Adam lifted his glasses from the side table and stuck them on Devon's nose.

"Your clothes and backpack are in the closet. You won't be hitting the books any time soon, though."

"Why'm I strapped down?"

"We've got two IV's—intravenous lines—running into you. One for meds and the other for blood. You got pretty anemic."

"What's going on? What hospital?"

"Here on campus. You passed out and they called the ambulance. The doc here'll explain everything."

I rolled Devon over to the bed's edge so Adam could free the bottom sheet. It was wringing wet.

Devon took in this latest eye-opener. "I peed the bed?"

"No worries there—you've got a catheter in," Adam reassured him. "To track your fluids, keep your kidneys working right."

We finished up our bed-making business and Devon closed his eyes, as though relishing the coolness. Adam reached to unstrap his arms.

"Go easy now." Then to me, "You want me to stay while you two chat?"

"Yeah, make sure I don't get too technical." I pulled up my chair. "Not too sleepy to talk a bit, Devon?"

"No, I wanna know."

"Well, you got real sick real quick. It'll take you a while to get back on top." I kept my words slow, made sure he was taking them in. "You have a fever. And you lost a lot of blood."

"Where?"

"In your bowel."

"Infection?"

"That may be part of it—we're not sure yet."

"What else then?"

"Devon, there's a tumour in your bowel. We need to take a piece of it, and then see if it can be cut out."

"Cancer?"

“We won’t know till the surgeons take a piece. But it’s possible.”

“Who knows I’m here?”

“I talked to your mom, she’s on her way here. But her plane’s delayed. She’ll call me as soon as she knows the new schedule. But I got her okay to go ahead with the surgery. You were too out of it to give your okay.”

The following morning, the surgeons confirmed what we had strongly suspected—a cancerous growth in the small bowel wall. They were able to remove what looked like the whole tumour, along with several inches of healthy appearing small intestine on each side. The attending surgeon, Judy, called me an hour later.

“Just got the report from Path, John. Non-Hodgkin’s—large cell. Pretty aggressive looking.”

Devon was still sleepy that evening when I checked in on him, but he was resting comfortably. His mother was due to arrive within the hour.

“You up for talking some more?”

“Yeah. What did those surgeons find?”

“It is cancer, Devon. But it looks like it hasn’t spread. And they were able to cut the whole thing out.”

He closed his eyes for a long moment, then reopened them. “What now?”

“We need to give you strong drugs. To make sure it doesn’t come back.”

“Cancer drugs?”

“Right.”

“My dad got them. They didn’t work.”

“What kind of cancer did he have?”

“Lymphoma. I was still a kid. Mom knows a lot more about it.”

I couldn't stop the flicker in my gaze. Devon picked up on it fast.

"That's it, isn't it? I've got what he got."

"Yes, Devon, you have. But there are different kinds. And chemo usually works really well …"

"What are my chances? Straight poop. 'M I going to die, like him?"

"I don't think so, Devon. The odds are better than even that you'll come through this. I'm just not going to promise you a hundred percent."

"A gamble, though, right? Like pulling straws. So what if I said, no way? I'm not going through with that shit?"

"That'd be real bad news, Devon. I would do everything I could to persuade you. Because chemo treatment gets better all the time—'specially in young guys like you."

"My dad drew the short straw."

"Tell me about your dad."

Tears pricked at his eyelids. "The drugs didn't work."

"How long ago, Devon?"

"I was a kid—six maybe. I'm twenty-one now."

"Fifteen years—that's a long time in our line of work. How old was he, you know?"

"Forty. Had his big four-o in the hospital. Mom said it was like he hung on for it."

"Some folks do—for an important date."

There was silence between us. His tears were flowing freely. I was glad to see he wasn't holding back. There are a lot of tears to cry at times like this—but male college students are mostly too macho to let them come. I hunted around for tissues, then grabbed a wad of toilet paper from the bathroom. “Unused, I promise.”

Devon snorted a giggle mingled with snot. A booger threatened to drop on my outstretched arm. He grabbed the tissue and blew hard.

“I’ll need to get hold of your dad’s records. You know where he got treated?”

“Boston. Mass General.”

“You remember anything about it?”

“It’s real vague. But my mom’s told me a lot. I wanted to know …”

“Talking about it’s good. A lot of folks can’t.”

“They never said it ran in families.”

“Lymphoma’s not one of the usual suspects. But some families get more than their fair share. They’re finding these genes now—I’ll read up on the latest studies.”

“I want to know. Everything.”

“You got it.”

“What’s going to happen? My hair gonna fall out?”

“Yes, Devon, I’m sorry. A side effect of the drugs—something I’m sure you don’t want, but we haven’t found how to prevent. It’ll grow back, promise—peach fuzz, like a baby’s.” I grinned briefly, then, “This whole thing’s a nightmare, right? Got to be wondering how you’ll make it through. But you will.”

“So what else? Warts on my nose?”

“Maybe a few on your fingers. You’ll be sick to your stomach, too, and it’ll be hard keeping your weight on. We’ll have to check your blood a lot—these drugs do some funny things.”

"Holy crap."

"Holy crap is right. But it's not forever."

"So how long am I going to be holed up here?"

"A few weeks."

"Shit, I'm s'posed to graduate next month. Gotta tell 'em at school."

"I'll talk with your dean, Devon. They make exceptions if you've kept your grades up."

"They're up there. Been planning on grad school—anthropology. My dad dug up a lot about where we came from—he went back four generations. Figured it was Senegal."

"Looks like the gods are telling you to take a break, Devon. But no reason you can't get right back on track. I'll chase up your dad's records, do my own research—about lymphoma and families."

"What happens when I get out?"

"Short breaks, then back for more of the same. Six courses in total. These are strong drugs, and you'll need to stay in hospital each time. But you're young, so it'll be easier."

"What if it's still there?"

"There's a high chance it won't be, Devon. Your kind of cancer grows fast, then it shrinks just as quick. I'll tell you a story. When I started training forty years ago, specialists were leery about ever stopping treatment. Couldn't get their heads around the idea—like with AIDS today. We had a patient with lymphoma, twenty-five when I knew her. She'd been taking chemo since she was eighteen.

"My very first clinic, she told me, 'Enough already—this chemo's messing with my social life.' I queried my prof about it. 'Never stopped anyone's treatment,' he told me. 'Maybe it's time, though—if we haven't cured her yet, I guess we never will.'

"She stopped treatment altogether that day. I looked after her my whole fellowship and went to her wedding. She'll be bouncing grandkids on her knee about now."

A tap at the door. Adam was back. "Sorry to interrupt you folks. But I've got more pain meds, Devon. Then I'll pull your cath."

He tugged on a pair of plastic gloves, pushed his syringe into the end of the IV then eased back the bedclothes. Devon looked down as the nurse untied his pajama strings.

"Jeez, tubes in my arms, in my gut, in my dick. And you guys shaved me clean!"

"No big deal getting this sucker out. One less thing to deal with."

As Adam finished up, the door swung open and a tall, middle-aged Black woman entered. She crossed the room swiftly, stretched out her arms. Devon scooched over and she eased down beside him, then paused to swing back around.

"Is one of you Devon's doctor? I'm his mom, Doreen Leonard."

"That'd be me. Adam here is his nurse."

She grasped each of our outstretched hands in turn.

"I'm sorry we're meeting in this situation, Mrs. Leonard. But your son's doing real well. I told you on the phone about the surgery, and we're all set to get his chemo started."

She twisted back around to her son. "Dev, the doctor's right—about the cancer, and it needing treatment right off. I told him—do what all it takes."

"He wants Dad's records, Mom. Gonna look up about lymphoma and families."

"I've got your first chemo ready, Devon, okay?" Adam intervened.

"Holy shit, no frigging peace around here!"

Devon's mother bumped her nose against his. "That's hospitals, Dev. Places of restful repose? Not!"

"Sorry, Devon. But we need to get things started right away."

Adam was easing the tube from Devon's stomach when I showed up for morning rounds. I had unearthed several papers about lymphoma in families.

"You'll be good for something solid soon," the nurse told him. "Not burgers and fries yet, though, more like apple sauce and Jell-O. Gently does it."

His mother roused herself from where she had been sacked out on the couch. She moved to the other side of the bed as I pulled up my chair.

"Mrs. Leonard, Devon handled his first chemo just great. And it looks like the bleeding inside has stopped."

"We talked a bunch last night. Thanks for squaring with him, not holding anything back."

"He quizzed me pretty hard. Devon, I promised I'd get the latest scoop. I've got a good bit of it here."

"Just the short version right now," Devon said.

"Well, it happens more in families than tossing a coin. It's early days, but they're finding genes that probably trigger the cancer."

"Like the ones Dad passed on to me?"

"It's not as simple as that. You ever hear tell of sickle cell disease?"

"Sure. A friend of mine in primary school, he had it."

"Right, it happens in Black families. Children inherit a gene from both Mom and Dad. But with cancer, it's different. We think the genes show up later and turn good cells into bad."

“Just as well you and Dad stopped with me, Mom.”

“The risk would still be awfully small, even if your mom had had ten of you,” I told him.

“So I drew the short straw. And I’ve gotta get on with it.”

“Another thing, though—real important. You may be a grown man, but you’re still a kid to me. And you need to know that chemo works a whole lot better when a body is young and fit. We don’t know why exactly, so that’s something you can research.”

“Doctoral thesis, maybe.”

“Could be. The big thing, though—whatever caused this thing, we’re gonna deal with it. I’m making you my special project.”

“It’s pretty scary, Doc.”

“Listen, Devon,” his mom intervened. “I’m scared too, but I’m not about to lose the other main man in my life.”

“You told me one time Dad’s cancer just laughed at the chemo, then kept on growing till it killed him. What if mine’s the same? I got half his genes.”

“And you got the other half from me. I’m fit as a fiddle—and I won’t see fifty again. You’re half your dad’s age when he passed, too. The doc told you that’s big.”

“Yeah. It’s just—like father, like son.”

“No, Dev, not like father, like son. I used to wonder where you came from—till I realized no two people could have those weird ears.”

“Yeah, I sure didn’t take after him most ways. I’m no jock.”

“Your dad had you all set to star in his Little Leagues team, dreamed of making the World Series. Till you couldn’t figure if you were a leftie or a rightie.”

“Still not sure.”

“Remember how proud he was when you caught your first fish. Big old five-year-old and you couldn’t stop bawling about how that hook had to be hurting.”

“I guess I was a disappointment.”

“Noo, Dev. He knew how smart you were. Knew those weren’t his genes—he hardly graduated high school. Had plenty of smarts, mind, just not your kind.”

“Guess so.”

“And he wasn’t all jock. You were always a hugger, but when you turned five, he declared too much cuddling would make you a sissy. I told him, ‘No way, hugs toughen you up!’ He never brought it up again. The night before I took him into hospital, that last time, you were wedged up between us in the bed.”

“And I can roll the sides of my tongue up, just like him.”

“Yup. I could spend my life trying, and never manage it!” She moved in closer on the bed beside her son, wrapped an arm around his shoulders. “Yeah, you got half your dad’s genes, Dev. But you’re not him. You’re not your dad.”

DUI

"I'm not letting you out of my sights till you're ninety-three in the shade."

I met Damien in the Intensive Care Unit—or rather, re-met him. He had ended up there after being arrested at 6.30 pm on a rainy Friday, the day before his twentieth birthday, on a charge of being drunk and disorderly while speeding his truck helter-skelter down Northwest 13th Street just north of the university. A police patrol car had spotted him as he ran a red light at University and 13th Street on three tires and a tire rim, skidded wildly to his right, mounted the curb, slid across the sidewalk, narrowly missed three pedestrians, a skateboarder, and the front of the Asian Fusion restaurant, and finally came to rest in a head of steam and a hedge of azaleas.

Smoke was rising from the engine when the first police officer jerked the driver's door open. Damien was slumped over the wheel, to all appearances sleeping off a late-afternoon binge. He made incoherent noises as the policeman tried to rouse him. After a second officer arrived, they concluded there was no immediate danger of the car going up in flames. To be on the safe side they summoned a fire engine and Billy's Towing from the nearby Shell garage to deal with the wreck, then together lifted Damien into the back of their patrol car. Ten minutes later, they were wheeling him into the Shands Emergency Room, strapped onto a gurney and with his hands cuffed behind his back.

But the two police officers were starting to have doubts. There had been a notable lack of the combativeness that most drunks display when roused from a post-binge slumber. Added to that, there was no obvious whiff of alcohol fumes. The senior nurse, whose job it was to triage each newcomer to her ER, stuck Damien well down on the priority list, assuming he was just another drunk who could be left to sleep it off for a while. But by the time one of the busy residents got around to examining him, Damien was beginning to stir, and the doctor noticed that he was barely moving his left side. On closer inspection, he thought he could detect clonus—an involuntary repetitive spasm—in his left ankle when he tested his reflexes. These repetitive involuntary muscle contractions usually indicate some kind of injury to the brain.

"We need a CAT scan *stat*," the resident told the staff nurse. "And get a tox screen as well as a blood alcohol level. Then we'll need Neurology to see him as soon as he's through in X-ray."

An hour later, the blood test confirmed that alcohol was not the problem. There wasn't a trace. Meanwhile Damien was under the CAT scanner, still pretty much out of it but beginning to roll around and mess up the images on the screen. The X-ray technician was having a hard time getting clear pictures, but she knew nobody was about to tranquilize him, given Damien's quite uncertain diagnosis. She phoned the on-call radiologist.

"Are you still in house? Can you take a look at these pictures and see if we've got enough? They don't want us to sedate this guy."

The attending radiologist had been packing his briefcase in his office in the next corridor when he got the call. He took a quick look at Damien, then at the slices of fuzzy brain images she had already obtained.

"You've got enough here to see there's no hemorrhage. And he's not herniating." (Meaning his upper brain wasn't getting squeezed downwards and putting potentially fatal pressure on his brain stem which controls breathing and circulation). "But I think there's something taking up space in his right cerebral cortex. It's not big, but it could be a tumour."

An hour later Damien was in a bed in our PICU on the neurosurgery service. He had received a large dose of intravenous Decadron to reduce any brain swelling, as well as Dilantin, an anti-seizure drug. The neurosurgeons had rightly surmised that Damien had suffered an epileptic seizure in his truck, and that he was still in a post-ictal state—the normal recovery phase that follows a seizure—when the police caught up with him. The PICU staff had called me, too. It was more of a courtesy at this stage—the suggestion of the attending neurosurgeon now that the possibility of a brain tumour had come up. We might be needed later if this was confirmed.

When I heard the name—Damien Ramirez—it set off a faint bell in my memory. "D'you have any medical history on him?" I asked the resident on the phone. "Anything more than what you've told me?"

"Nope. They haven't got a hold of any family yet. And he's in no fit state to tell us much of anything."

"But you say he's twenty, or will be tomorrow?"

"Right."

"I'll be right up to see him. I think I know this guy. In the meantime, can you call down to medical records, see if they can pull up anything on him? It's probably been ten years, so I don't think there will be anything on the computer."

Nowadays, most hospitals can locate a patient's old hospital records instantly on the computer, but this is a quite recent advance. Unneeded records more than five years old would likely be gathering dust in thick charts in the basement. Damien was still sleepy when I pulled up a chair at his bedside, but he was starting to mumble, and his nurse had got him to suck a little tea through a straw. I only needed to take one look at him. He was a good bit older, but he was the same guy I had come to know very well more than ten years back. Just in case I needed it, I was clasping the thick and dusty chart that a records clerk had uncovered for me in a basement stack.

One of our hospital security guards was sitting in the window glancing through the paper, but I knew his charge didn't pose any risks to anyone. I put a hand on Damien's shoulder and shook him gently.

"Hiya, Damien. You remember me?"

He turned his head and half-opened his eyes. There was a look of instant recognition.

"Hi, Doc." Slurry, but clear enough.

I had known him since he was a toddler with newly diagnosed acute lymphoblastic leukemia, and seen him through three years of chemotherapy, then five more years of follow-up appointments. There hadn't been a single setback, so at that point I had decided I didn't need to make any more clinic appointments. His family lived locally, and I continued to get Christmas cards as well as other reassuring news about him. I seemed to remember hearing about him starting as a freshman at our university a year or so ago.

"Damien, are you in school here?"

"Yeah." He looked around him, then back at me. "What happened to me?"

"You had an accident. Crashed your truck. You remember anything about it?"

He looked startled. "No. I don't remember a thing. Jeez, my head hurts."

"We'll get you something. It looks like you passed out, maybe had a seizure. But you're okay. We just have to figure out why it happened to you."

The next day, Damien was fully able to cooperate during the MRI scan of his brain that would give us a clear look at what was going on in there. It confirmed what the radiologist had suspected: a tumour about two centimetres square was sitting right in the middle of his right cerebral cortex. It was impossible to tell if it was cancerous or not; only an operation would yield that information. Second tumours crop up in about ten percent of children who are cured of their first cancer. Those who have had radiation of any sort are probably at higher risk, and Damien had indeed had his brain irradiated. It had been standard procedure at that time to prevent the spread of leukemia into his nervous system.

By the time I got to talk to Damien again, his mother was sitting at his bedside. We recognized each other at once and exchanged hugs.

"I'm very sorry we're meeting again in these circumstances, Mrs. Ramirez. I hear they have him scheduled for surgery tomorrow."

"Yes. He seems fine now, but he doesn't remember anything about what happened."

"Damien, this tumour looks like it's pretty small still, and they can only see it in that one place. There's a good chance they can get it all out without any damage to you."

"I'm real weak in my arm and leg, Doc. My left one." His speech was almost back to normal. "Will that get better?"

"It'll take some work with the physical therapist. But you're a young guy, no reason why you can't be skipping about in no time."

Damien was in the operating room for five hours the next day. Shortly after six in the evening, the pediatric neurosurgeon called me.

"Hey, this thing shelled out very nicely. It's an astro (*astrocytoma*), and looks low-grade. I don't think we'll be needing you guys."

Histological grading is a crucial part of the assessment of all brain tumours. A low grade indicates a low degree of malignancy. Such tumours, though cancerous, can usually be cured by surgery alone if they can be safely removed. Things were looking up for Damien. Three days later he was up on crutches, although shaky and favoring his right side. He summoned a little scatological humour

"Hey, I managed a BM today, Doc. Probably that enema they gave me!"

"Good job, buddy. And I heard the final word. They got the whole thing out, and you're not going to need any more chemo. But I'm not letting you out of my sights until you're ninety-three in the shade."

Lumps

How much easier to shield him from this vital piece of his training

The first outpatient clinic of the new year, I saw only three patients myself. Curtis, one of our oncology fellows, saw the rest. But it felt like I did my share.

Five-year-old Jimmy was in for his check-up, a year out from a bone marrow transplant to try to cure his refractory leukemia. He had been fine, his mother April told me, but there was a sad look on her face. She was thirty and had three others under ten. I sat beside her waiting for more, and she finally blurted out that their dad had just left their eleven-year marriage. She had no money, no transport, and had moved in with her sister forty miles away. Medicaid had paid for her bus fare today.

Jimmy's leukemia had been slow to respond initially, I remembered. But fortune had smiled, his older sister Becky was a full HLA-match, meaning their genetic make-up was so similar it was unlikely that Jimmy would reject Becky's bone marrow cells. So we had gone straight to bone marrow transplant after he had struggled into an initial remission. He had then sailed through this most extreme of treatments and was growing more boisterous with every visit. The mass of dark curls bounced on his scalp as he jumped onto the table.

But there was something new today—the unequivocal swelling of his spleen below his left ribcage. I went to check his blood count in our small outpatient lab. His white cell count was 51,000, almost ten times normal, and his platelet count 48,000, about twenty-five percent of normal. It's a sure sign of trouble—you could call it an oncology saw—when your white count is higher than your platelet count. I peered down the microscope at his blood film and saw it at once: an almost solid wall of leukemia cells. I closed my eyes for several long moments, then grabbed Tom, one of our two clinic nurses.

“Jimmy’s relapsed. Can you free yourself up for a few minutes?”

“Sure.’

Tom followed me back to Jimmy’s exam room, where he busied the little guy with an auto magazine. I watched as Jimmy ran busy fingers over the racing green sweep of the center-fold Jaguar XK.

“That’s the one I’m going to get!”

I pulled my chair in close to April, held her eye, took in the gathering look of dread. No way I could break the news gently.

“April, Jimmy’s leukemia is back.”

She held a long breath before the sobs shook loose.

“Mom’s crying,” Jimmy said to Tom. “She cries a lot.”

A long time later, I left them to hurry to Alyssa’s room. An elegant first-year undergraduate, she had come under my care for a highly malignant sarcoma arising out of her pelvis. She had already gone through surgery, but they could only remove part of the cancer. So we had followed swiftly with our best chemotherapy, while the radiation oncologists had doled out daily doses of intensive radiation aimed directly at the cancer. This potent combination had achieved a tenuous remission and after a long convalescence Alyssa was able to resume some of her classes. But she knew all too well after quizzing me that the chances of her being cured were always slim.

Now this unscheduled visit. Rachel, our other clinic nurse, had alerted me that Alyssa had been retching up what was left of her stomach contents ever since she had arrived half an hour earlier. A student buddy of hers was sitting beside her gurney holding onto the kidney bowl. She got up quickly when I came in.

“D’you want me to leave, Doctor?”

"No, no, you stay put." I knew her from earlier visits, and knew she was a great support to her friend. It was good to have a female chaperone, too, and not to have to bring Rachel in. I turned my attention to Alyssa. "You hurting a lot?"

Alyssa nodded mutely, then managed to pull herself up to hug me. It felt like she clung on a good bit more than in her usual brief embraces. At her clinic visit four weeks earlier, I had been worried about the size of some of the lymph nodes in her groin. At least one of them had doubled its dimension.

"They've gotten bigger, Doc."

She had been all too aware of my worries at her last visit. I avoided probing her belly, not wanting to set off more retching. I let my fingers run gently over her groin. Several other glands had now grown to an abnormal size.

"You're right, Alyssa. We don't really need another scan."

"We gave it our best shot, I guess." She gestured urgently to her friend for the kidney bowl. After a further dry heave, she dropped back full length on the exam table. "Maybe we could try that last lot of chemo you gave me again. Seemed like it did something to slow the sucker down."

I felt a tightening in my throat at her defiant attitude. I didn't trust myself to respond at once. I let the quiet build a little, then reached to take her hand.

"We could certainly give it a try, Alyssa. Maybe you want to think things over some, talk to your mom and dad. Meanwhile, I'll give you something to settle your stomach down." I smiled at her friend. "I'm sorry, I've forgotten your name."

"Taylor."

"Taylor, can you stay with Alyssa for a bit?"

"Sure, yeah. I'm not going anywhere."

Alyssa directed her gaze at her friend. “Thanks, girl.” Then to me, “Doc, it’d be good if you could call my folks first. Then I’ll talk with them once they know what’s happening. I already kind of prepared them.”

“I’ll do it right away, Alyssa.”

The three of us sat quietly together for a few more minutes. Alyssa’s nausea seemed to be settling. I excused myself, knowing there was already a backlog of patients building, even though Curtis had been steadily working his way through them, barely having to summon me for advice. As I left the exam room, I almost bumped into Cheryl—Robert’s mother.

“He’s ready for his chemo this week, John.”

She had been comfortable using my first name from the first time I’d first met her. Very much a woman who took charge. But her teenage son had been giving her as good as he got. Robert had an osteosarcoma that had started out in his left femur but had already spread to his lungs when we first saw him two months earlier. Last week he had refused more chemotherapy, but judging from her confident words it seemed like his mom had persuaded him.

“Can we get on up to Admissions?” she continued. “Robert’s ready to go.”

Her husband appeared at her side, looking tense. Not for the first time, I felt them both pushing on me, just like they were pushing on their fifteen-year-old.

“Let me just take a look at Robert, okay? I won’t be able to get up to the ward till this evening to check him out.”

He was already in his exam room, his once strapping athlete’s body seeming to shrink into itself. He had gone through a thoracotomy last month, only two months after his initial major surgery to remove the primary cancer from his femur. This latest surgery had been the second one in what was to me a very questionable attempt to fish out the metastases that had spread to both his lungs. Once a cancer has spread to distant parts the chances of catching the bolting horse were slim to none.

"Can't I wait a while?" Robert started in as soon as he saw me. "I've not eaten anything in forever, and I'm real weak."

Cheryl jumped in. "You know this is the right thing to do, Robert. We've been through this already. You're not going to get any better without it."

I caught her stricken look, the tears glistening close behind.

"Well, there's no right or wrong," I murmured, already knowing my words were falling on deaf ears as far as Cheryl and her husband were concerned. Robert stayed silent, and I knew his dad wasn't about to side with him against his wife. Not for the first time, I reflected on this impossible but all too familiar situation—a teenager with incurable cancer, still a minor in the law's eyes, directly opposed to his parents' wishes. More often than not, I felt myself siding with the patient.

"Robert, let's give this a try," I answered him. "Your mom's right. If it's going to work, it's far better not to delay things anymore."

His eyes, then his head, drooped in silent acquiescence, subjugate to my words. His tongue licked furtively at a single boulder tear rolling slowly down his left cheek. I felt my own tears welling up as I left him and his parents to call the oncology ward to confirm his room was ready. I glanced at my watch: four-forty already, and I'd seen a total of three patients. Curtis emerged from the one other exam room that was still occupied.

"Well done, Curtis," I greeted him. "Looks like you've done more that your fair share today."

"It's been fine, John. I didn't have to deal with any of the problems you've had."

I reflected on how he would have handled my three patients and their families, and how much easier it was, maybe for both of us, to shield him from this vital piece of his training. When all the staff had headed home, I sat and breathed, shook with cumulative grief for Jimmy, and Alyssa, and Robert, and for each of their families. My whole body, mind, and spirit had been engaged today. Next week, I would be certain to take Curtis along on this journey. Or maybe I would just step back and leave him to see those few tough cases, while I kept the rest of the clinic happily flowing along. It was the only way to learn—on the job. And either you could hack it, or you'd be best to take up a less demanding line of work.

Part Three

Remembering

Connective Tissue

'Your voice is his. Your gestures, too.'
So his fleshless ash lives on in me.

After Dad's Cremation, 1991

A month after retiring from the University of Florida in 2007, two letters came in the mail from England: my birth certificate (*February 23rd, 1942*), replacing the one I had lost somewhere on my travels, and my final pension award from Newcastle-on-Tyne. Newcastle is not only home to the British Pension Office but also the city of my father's death sixteen years earlier. This full life cycle, tucked into two envelopes resting in my mailbox one upon the other, sent me off on a journey of reminiscence.

In October 1941, my mother turned up for her weekly Women's Institute fitness class in the village church hall. Mummy looked all set to deliver me into the world, but she reassured her friend Christine who expressed concern about her doing Jumping Jacks so far along in her pregnancy: "The doctor says it's fine. Might even move things along a bit—after all, this will be my fourth."

The doctor being my dad, *aka* Dick, whose word on any health issue was law in High Bickington and the surrounding Devonshire hamlets. I have this conversation on good authority, because I met up with Christine seventy years later on the eve of her hundredth birthday. Once she had figured out who I was, she recounted a favorite memory—of me bouncing up and down inside thirty-nine-year-old Mummy at thirty-six weeks, while Mummy herself bounced up and down to the rhythm of *Run, Rabbit, Run*, which was currently topping the hit parade.

I was born at term, so I calculate those two gametes that created my very own first zygote came together on May 29th, 1941, my sister Jane's second birthday:

Dick's sprightly young sperm flying solo through Mummy's fimbrial folds to pierce a single blushing ovule. They say conceiving is more fun than the delivering, but I never got to ask either Mummy or Dick their opinion on that issue.

They were living in my paternal grandmother's house in Golders Green in North London at the time, while Dick finished his surgical internship under William Girling Ball, Dean of Barts medical school. I like to picture the two of them cozied up like canned sardines right beneath squadrons of dog-fighting Spitfires and Messerschmitts. So began my replication towards the thirty-seven-trillion-cell being I would become thirty-eight weeks on. In the meantime I spent those blissful months of womb life tuning into the soothing rhythms of Mummy's placental blood-lullaby.

By delivery time—a mercifully swift one for both Mummy and me—the thunderclap of bombs was replaced by the evening chorus of blackbirds and wood pigeons in the hawthorn hedges of rural Devon. Dick had bought a three-hundred-square-mile practice in the village of High Bickington, a Saxon settlement dating from 700 A.D. sandwiched between Exmoor to the north and Dartmoor to the south, where Conan Doyle's hellish *Hound of the Baskervilles* had been wont to roam and ravage. Our home sat astride two country lanes that converged to form a long straight hill up to the village. In time-honoured English custom, the house had at some time been given a name—*Dobbs*—though the origin and significance of this are lost. The ancient pear tree in our back garden still bore fruit when we lived there and the seventeenth-century well yielded its spring water year-round.

I was born in my parents' bed, with Dick and Nurse Lumney—an old flame from medical student days Dick brought along for all Mummy's confinements—in attendance. He may have looked approvingly upon his firstborn son after fathering three girls, but my first day was not without trauma. He had no truck with paragraph five of the Hippocratic oath—*I will not use the knife ... but will withdraw in favour of such men as are engaged in this work.* So at one hour of extrauterine life my father circumcised me on our dining room table—a heavy slab of 1920s oak on which I am right now leaning my elbows as I write, flinching at the memory.

He brought to the task a special mix of *sangfroid* and *rituel*, while paying more attention to Nurse Lumney than to the suffering willy on the end of his scalpel. Circumcisions were bread-and-butter stuff and he tackled the task without the benefit of any local anesthetic. True to most doctors of the day, he considered newborn nerve endings—boy ones anyway—too immature to feel the knife. Today we know our sensory network is finely honed from well before birth. Mothers quickly learn to soothe their unborn babies with lullabies as soon as they start stretching their limbs within their cozy bedchambers.

Mummy slept through my *bris* blissfully unaware of my agony as I pined for the blessed balm of her nipple. A surgeon *manqué*, Dick used that sturdy oak table for other more substantial procedures, from setting eldest sister Elizabeth's fractured radius, sustained after crashing off her bike on Ebberley Hill as she cycled up to the village, to injecting the newly available penicillin into the cerebrospinal fluid of a toddler he suspected of meningitis. Dick was the only person for miles about with a car—a racing green MG Midget that dated from the earliest 1936 prototype, which he drove with roof down both summer and winter. The villagers spoke of him as a fine doctor but a devil of a driver.

After completing his early-morning house calls in the surrounding villages he would roar into the driveway fronting our house with a screech of brakes and a scattering of gravel, barely avoiding his lovingly tended boxwood hedge. He would stride into his morning clinic through our back door hauling off his massive leather driving gloves. It was the same backdoor that his patients would already have entered, each one triggering a bell peel through the rest of the house. Two rows of farmers and labourers would be perched with their wives and children amid a mix of eagerness and dread on the benches under the windows awaiting his ministrations.

For carrying out his physical exams Dick had two curtains on castors that Mummy had sewn and assembled. But there were few secrets in the village's butcher or baker shop because he never lowered his voice below a bark. One morning when I was around four, I succeeded in easing the door to his clinic far enough open to get a clear view of the scene unfolding before me. A sight worthy of undiminished memory: a comely fourteen-year-old girl was seated naked to the waist on the examining table while Dick declaimed his store of home remedies for period and growing pains. Her mother was struggling to keep up, while her daughter looked utterly at home with the attention—if a mite chilled. Perhaps she'd grown accustomed to such early-morning exposure to her fatherly doctor.

Dick had constructed pine shelves on three of the clinic walls to hold his multitude of medicinals, giving loving attention to each perfectly tooled edge and elegantly engineered dowel. He stored his *placebos* in amber-coloured jars, mounted with ground-glass stoppers and labeled in his calligraphic scroll with names like *Nux vomica, Chlorina liquida, Gentiana spp., Camphora officianalis*, reminiscent of an eighteenth-century apothecary's shop. He dispensed these seemingly identical white powders and poisonous-looking potions with a customary flourish, to the obvious awe of his clientele, always insisting that they be consumed in wine glasses.

Was this last injunction ever followed? Hard to imagine these unworldly country folk being able to lay their hands on a single crystal goblet between them. But his awesome authority surely served as an even more potent placebo, whatever the presenting complaint—asthma or angina, chickenpox or collywobbles. In the memoir he wrote shortly before his death there is a verbatim account of one grateful patient, the broad Devonshire brogue readily detectable:

"You bin very good to I, Dr. Pole. I brought a big fat duck for 'ee. Us'd like another bottle of that there brown medicine, Dr. Pole, thank 'ee kindly. 'Ere be your 'alf-crown."

The clinic's remaining wall space was adorned with watercolours and pen-and-ink sketches, for Dick was an artist as much as a medical scientist. Not only was he adept with the paintbrush and fine-line marker but he could construct a three-story doll house, glue together the intricate parts of a fully working model engine and perform magic tricks with impenetrable sleight-of-hand. His espaliers of roses and apple trees ranged along the garden walls in glorious symmetry, while his beehives won prizes every August at the Exmoor agricultural and livestock show.

Dick also found time and occasion to indulge his fleshly appetites through frequent trysts with our two maids (whether *en solo* or *ménage a trois* I never found out). His younger women patients were also far from immune from his advances. He eventually came a cropper after a passionate affair with a mother of two I'll call Erica. When Mummy demanded he break it off or she'd head home to Grandma with us four children, he made some effort to put an end to his philandering. Erica promptly threatened to report him to the General Medical Council unless he left Mummy and married her. This brought him within a hair's breadth of losing his medical license, and after several trial separations Mummy divorced him and moved us all sixty miles up the west coast of England to Weston-super-Mare in the county of Somerset, where her parents lived on the edge of the Bristol Channel.

Right after the divorce Dick married Erica. At five years old I had no warning of his imminent departure. For the next sixteen years there was not a moment's connection between me and my father. His name was barely mentioned at home and the only trace of him was a photo—"Dick and Doreen, October, 1933"—taken in a moment of honeymoon bliss. They are reclining close together in the heather of a Scottish Highlands hillside, he sporting a meerschaum pipe and Mummy nursing a picnic hamper. Did such moments of marital bliss make it through to my conception? Or was I the offspring of a momentary reconciliation after ever more shenanigans—a brief blip in the downward spiral of a marriage already dead?

And was the sixteen-year silence between him and me of Mummy's choosing or his? I never asked Mummy directly, but I have a strong hunch my grandmother's acrimony towards Dick played a decisive part, given his minimal financial support of us four children. Mummy was almost totally dependent on Grandma throughout my childhood. One welcome irony of this whole debacle was that I was awarded a full scholarship to Epsom College boys-only boarding school from aged twelve to eighteen. The college had been endowed in 1855 and began life as The Royal

Medical Benevolent College, with the express goal of "providing the orphans of medical families with free housing, clothing and schooling." The college's medical foundation saw me as an abandoned child—essentially an orphan. So not only was I a fully paid-up foundationer but this benevolence lasted into my university years. When I won a Classics scholarship to Barts medical school (Dick's *alma mater*) the medical foundation went on to pay every penny of my six years of tuition.

I had one other small but memorable connection to Dick during my schooldays. Just before my first term at Epsom College Mummy brought down a battered trunk from the attic to ferry my possessions on the train from home to school and back. On it were two address labels, one bearing Dick's address at University College in London, where he had obtained his B.Sc. in Physiology, and the other with his subsequent address at Barts medical college. They became a talisman of sorts for me during those years.

The sixteen-year silence between us was broken at last during my third year at medical school with a three-minute phone call from Dick inviting me to celebrate my twenty-first birthday with him and his family. At 7.30pm sharp on February 23rd, 1963, I shook hands with my father on the steps of the Odeon Cinema in Leicester Square. He was a man I had no reason to recognize, having no visual memory of him beyond that thirty-year-old honeymoon photo. There followed handshakes with wife Erica and my two step-siblings, after which we sat in a row in the Grand Circle of the palatial cinema and watched four hours of *Lawrence of Arabia*. The total silence between us seemed longer than the decade and a half preceding it.

But now we were connected once more and I spent many weekends with him, medicine being a natural bond between us. He would tell me tales of other doctors in our family tree, none of whom I had ever heard of. Among my medical forebears was my great-grandfather, John Nicholson, who graduated from Edinburgh Medical College in the 1870's, then traveled as a ship's surgeon from Penrith in Cumbria to Benalla in Victoria. He attended the notorious bush ranger and bank robber, Ned Kelly, and was alleged on one occasion to have removed nineteen bullets from various gang members while never revealing the gang's whereabouts to the police.

I had always thought my decision to become a physician was inspired by Mummy's early death from cancer, but perhaps there is a doctoring gene passed down through the generations. On the face of it, I was ill-suited to my chosen profession, given my early passion towards the humanities matched by an equally intense aversion for the sciences. After Mummy's death, I moved to my Uncle Ken's home in Yorkshire—Mummy's brother and another doctor. He did his level best to talk me out of following Dick and himself into the medical profession. As the sole doctor for three-thousand miners and their families in the coalmining district of Yorkshire, Uncle Ken was soured by his never-ending attendance at the deathbeds of these men, most victims in their thirties and forties to the "black lung" (as pneumoconiosis was popularly known). He would rouse me from bed in the early hours to hold vigil with him, no doubt seeing it as a deterrent to my misguided career ambitions. But I think it was these experiences that drew me late in my career to fulltime hospice work.

Dick's marriage to Erica ended in acrimony. She evicted him from the marital home one Christmas Eve and dumped his possessions on the doorstep of his clinic. She then took him to the High Court of Justice where it was decreed that "the marriage be dissolved by reason that the Respondent had treated the Petitioner with cruelty. The Commissioner orders the Respondent to pay the costs of his wife's suit." Dick claimed to not have the means to do so.

He worked on for several years in his single-handed practice in Guildford, the county town of Surrey in the heart of the stockbroker belt. To the utter bewilderment of his *Sassenach* patients, he would make his house calls wearing the kilt of his family clan—*Graham of Menteith*—complete with belt and buckle, horsehair sporran, dark kilt hose and garters and a prominently displayed *dirk*. He no longer conducted formal clinics and I rarely saw him field a phone call that called for his attendance. When I visited him, we would mostly spend our weekends at Farnham Sailing Club or at Kempton Park racecourse placing lavish bets on losers.

In time Dick retired with his third wife, Frances, Erica's children's former nanny, to the village of Milburn in Cumbria in the heart of Wordsworth's Lake District. He spent much of his time in thigh-high waders casting his elegant bamboo rods into the local tarn to hook many a delicious rainbow trout. For several years he joined me for New Year festivities while I was working at the Yorkhill Children's Hospital in Glasgow. *Hogmanay* was celebrated in grand style, with long lines outside the liquor stores throughout New Year's Eve. It was at one of these celebrations that I tried to get him talking about our disconnection throughout my childhood. We were both pretty liquored up and Dick saw my questioning as bitter recrimination. He took off home next morning, and this proved to be a final severing of all links between us: the second time in my life he had left me without so much as a goodbye.

Having outlived Mummy by fifty years, he died quickly from acute monoblastic leukemia—a rare illness in the old. He had himself admitted to the Freeman's Hospital in Newcastle-on-Tyne, where he challenged the interns with tests of his own concoction. My sister Jane phoned me at work at Shands Hospital where I was the attending pediatric oncologist. The call came through to our bone marrow transplant unit as I sat at the bedside of a seventeen-year-old girl who was also dying of refractory leukemia.

"They don't give him long," Jane told me. "Maybe a few weeks. But he's determined to get chemotherapy."

It was a measure of the distance that had opened between us that Dick made no attempt to contact me after his diagnosis, though he knew all about my quarter-century of close acquaintance with the very illness that had beset him. I shuddered at the thought of my eighty-seven-year-old father suffering through the rigours of intensive chemo, whose horrid toxicities I witnessed every day. I put in my own call to his hospital ward, only to find that he had died six hours earlier, lulled in the arms of merciful narcosis. I found out later that he had changed his will the night before his death, removing the names of five of his offspring including me, while naming as beneficiary only my sister Mary, who had kept in close touch with him during his declining years.

I stood in the nurses' station and wept for the unresolved issues between us, grieving the bitter way our patchwork fifty-year relationship had ended in one final burst of disconnection. Ayman, who was in the second year of his fellowship with us, wrapped his comforting Syrian arms around me, then took over my attending duties without a pause while I flew home to Cumbria for Dick's funeral. The next day I visited the ward in the Freeman's Hospital where my father had died. Judith, who nursed him through his last night on earth, talked to me with tears in her eyes: "He was hiding all his terror behind belligerence until I lulled him into slumber with a blessed infusion of morphine." At his cremation I was reunited with three generations of my family, including my two eighty-plus-year-old paternal aunts. Auntie Peggy, whom I had not seen for thirty years, told me: "Your voice is his. Your gestures too."

So his fleshless ash lives on in me, leaving me with lasting sadness—that we two human beings who had both chosen working lives committed to the healing of others, had so failed to mend the sad disconnect between our common tissue. Eighteen years on from his death, I have more compassion than anger toward him for his lifelong narcissism, petty cruelties, arrogance, and depravity—but can this amount to love? Mr. Rogers tells us, "You can love anyone if you know their story." I could claim I never really knew my father's story. But I've pieced together enough to have a strong sense of him as a deeply troubled man—one who could never face up to the hurts he had inflicted on his wives and children, and who knows how many others.

Despite his abandoning me twice without a word, he really wanted me as part of his life. To share times of fun and whoopee, good food and drink, and deep metaphysical conversation. For my part, I can feel not only affection but also awe toward him for all his skills and accomplishments as both multifaceted artist and medical scientist. Does this amount to love? The Greek word, *storge*, fits better—the two-way affection between father and son.

How did I avoid most of the pitfalls that devastated Dick's life and threatened to do the same to all those he professed to love? I know almost nothing about his early life and upbringing, so can't begin to judge how far they molded his personality and values. I do know it took me till I was thirty-six—a university professor, twelve years out from medical school, and the father of two adopted children who had just ended my first marriage—to acknowledge my own deep-seated emotional trauma. Trauma that I came to recognize was born primarily out of Dick's abandonment and Mummy's early death. It took me two years of skilled psychotherapy to begin to feel the lasting joy and purpose in life that has sustained me since.

An even harder question—what of Dick's fleshless ash lives on in me? I too have had a lifelong desire for knowledge and a strong creative streak (I pushed myself against the odds to rise high in my profession as a medical researcher, then late in my career came to espouse the arts over the sciences). I too am an extrovert, sometimes to the point of eccentricity (I used to run regular "playshops" for students and peers where we all dressed up in silly costumes and played children's party games). I too can admit to a potent sexuality, expressing itself in a lifelong hunger for intimacy and gratification (more than fulfilled in my marriage to Dorothy after a lifetime of searching).

On his eightieth birthday Dick told me, "The biggest mistake I made in my life was to fail profoundly in my marriage to your mother." He followed this up by writing in his memoir that "she was kindly and compassionate toward all with whom she came in contact … greatly loved, I would say revered … a wonderful wife and mother." Whenever I feel anger toward Dick for the largely self-inflicted screw-up he made of his life, these two affirmations—too little too late though they be— free up feelings in me akin to love.

Conkers and Nectarines

Breakfast
It was on just such a damp Somerset morning
she mounded porridge into a Blitz-evacuated bowl

Quick, 2002

Porridge has always been a comfort food for me. Like soft-boiled eggs, guarded by toy soldiers of hot buttered toast strips, or creamy mashed potatoes, baked macaroni pudding, and Tetley's tea brewed loose in the pot and served with milk (after the requisite five minutes of steeping). Food to resort to when I feel the need of the comfort my mother always gave me through my childhood. Porridge was integral to those Weston-super-Mare years. Mummy never let me out of the house for school, at least from the start of the Winter term until the end of the Easter term six months later, without making sure I coated my stomach with two platefuls of porridge, loaded with Lyle's golden syrup and milk—or cream, if those thirsty sparrows had left us any. Always the traditional Scottish Oats that could be left on a very low heat all night, never the quick Quaker Oats favoured today.

The glass milk bottles had aluminum tops, which we thought were made of silver. The milkman left them on our back stoop on his early-morning rounds. I never found out what time he came because I always slept the blissful sleep of a child. But the equally early-morning sparrows had ample time to peck through to where the cream accumulated at the top. I've never seen a hungry sparrow—they're among nature's survivors, like the crows. My porridge had to be glutinous enough for me to build castles that sagged in the middle as I worked my way in from the outer edge. I would flirt with the heat and always scald the roof of my mouth before setting off for St. Peter's preparatory school, especially if I was—habitually—running late. But the glow would light up my stomach as I sauntered—habitually—

the two miles from my back gate with my gang of dayboys, Traps (Mike Trapnell), Dates (John Davis), Sid (Anthony Ellis), and Joey (Anthony Ross). Who knows where their nicknames came from, but mine was easy enough—Guinea, short for Guinea Pig, the initials of my double-barreled surname. Were their stomachs glowing too, I would wonder but never check.

Weston was a seaside resort beloved of the pottery and steel foundry workers from the West Midlands *Black Country*, so named in early Victorian times for its dense layer of soot that covered everything from the coking, iron foundries, and thirty-foot-thick coal seam: Blake's dark satanic mills. Trainloads of trippers, as we nicknamed the tourists, would arrive on the first day of August for the prescribed two weeks of annual holiday. They would sit on rented deck chairs from morn till night, whatever the weather, and gaze out at Weston's far-distant sea, while their children rode up and down the sands on the donkeys—the Mager family's business since 1886.

No doubt drawn by its balmy offshore breezes, my maternal grandparents had retired to Weston from Swindon in Wiltshire, where they had made a pretty penny buying, doing up, and reselling shops and houses. On a clear day you could see right across this narrow strip of water to South Wales, the country of Mummy's forebears. While her family came from South Wales, my father's hailed from the south of Scotland, and I was raised in the south of England. Most of my adult life I've lived in the south of America and Canada, so I think of myself as a Southern Anglo-Celtic-American-Canadian. Who knows what other ethnic blood circulates inside?

Shortly after we had settled in Weston Mummy took my three elder sisters and me to visit my grandparents. I vividly remember spying on my grandpa as he lay in their double bed, although I was no more than five. I was quickly shooed out by the grown-ups, because this soon proved to be my grandfather's deathbed. How long he had been granted to enjoy his retirement home I don't know. But everyone denied later that I had been in the presence of death, so I must have asked about it a lot. Even today we keep our children well away from the presence of death, yet what a wonderful comfort it could be for our elders to spend their last moments with their grandchildren. Poet David Whyte has a delightful piece about his one-year-old son taking his very first steps on the gravestone of Ann Braithwaite, an early Quaker who had been buried in Hawkshead churchyard a century earlier. A reassuring symbol of the continuity of things: "…the lifting red socks, her exit to the world his entrance …"

Came the day, a year or two after we had left Devon, when we moved from St. Martin's, our home in a road with the mysterious name of Montpelier, a mile or two west to Ravenswood, 47 Bristol Road. It was a huge limestone house divided into two still-sizeable homes. The grander half was owned by John, a lawyer, and the glamorous Cora, his opera singer-wife who performed professionally in Bristol and no doubt at other exotic venues beyond my imagining. We now lived across the road from my grandma's house in Landemann Circus, much closer to Westcliff, my sisters' school, and to St Peter's, the school I would be attending once I turned seven.

Our home had always been filled to overflowing with Mummy's books, most of them moving with her from London where she had gained her MFA in literature at Bedford College in the late 1920s. I would often take them down in handfuls to browse through, no doubt looking vainly for interesting pictures, or playing games with her dog-eared Penguin paperbacks to see how many I could stack on end. But now was the time to move every one of them from old to new home: God forbid that a single well-thumbed page should be left behind. We knew no one with a car, so she and I tramped back and forth between houses while the girls were in school, hefting as high a pile of books as we could manage, along with bags of other treasures.

Soon after our move to Weston we took the paddle steamer "Ravenswood"—delighting that it had the same name as our new house—across the Bristol Channel to Newport on the Welsh coast, the home of Grandma Jackson's sister, my great-aunt Jessie. We picnicked in her back garden shaded from the August sunshine by ancient elms and beeches. Aunt Jessie gave me my first nectarine to eat—and my last till I spied them in the supermarket shortly after I moved to Cleveland more than thirty years later. I still get a thrill at buying a handful of nectarines at a time, although—perhaps like first kisses—they never taste as delectable as Aunt Jessie's.

I loved to get Mummy to myself, but I can count on my fingers the number of times I pulled it off. The demands of my three elder sisters, coupled with Mummy's unending domestic chores, made it hard for me to hold her full attention for more than a few minutes. So I learned early on the rewards of service. I would leap gleefully in response to her requests—and soon enough those of my sisters—up and down stairs to carry some small item from one of the bedrooms back down to the kitchen or drawing room.

But how especially prized were those Saturday morning shopping trips on the bus to Weston's town center, Mummy and I each toting a battered shopping bag down the High Street. Every shop was dedicated to a single item of commerce. The fishmonger and greengrocer swung down their awnings early in the morning, laying out with loving precision fresh fruits of land and sea. Mummy soon knew all these cheery and ruddy-faced shopkeepers by name. They would hawk their wares in the manner of Victorian street criers, proudly announcing the special offers of the day. Our final treat was a visit to the sweet shop next to our bus stop in The Boulevard. I could gaze on huge jars of humbugs and acid drops, lined up next to the licorice sticks, sherbet lemons, and jaw-breaking gobstoppers.

Sometimes I would have the agonizing luxury of deciding how to spend the last of my pocket money, though usually it was all gone by this stage of the week. But Mummy would always buy a large bar of Cadbury's chocolate for our after-Sunday-lunch treat (Cadbury's is a very old Quaker family, though I never recall any link being made to my later spiritual home). In summer we might venture down to the sea front for a magical six-inch stick of "rock" with the name Weston-super-Mare imprinted diagonally down the whole length of each succulent pink-and-white cylinder. Once on the bus, I would clutch my shopping bag on my knee, thigh-to-thigh with Mummy as the bus trundled around the corner and up the steep hill of Arundel Road and right onto Bristol Road to our stop at the top of

Montpelier. I was tired but blissed out. More than seventy years later, I smile every morning at her portrait by my computer, and her steadfast dark eyes and soft smile return my gaze.

Sometimes on a Saturday evening, we four children would gather in the drawing room around Mummy as she played "The Skye Boat Song" or "Loch Lomond" or "The White Cliffs of Dover." We would sing along until we were hoarse and ready to drop into bed. After I was safely tucked in, the grown-ups would sneak off to the *Hole in the Wall* pub, Mummy often accompanied by her off and-on-again boyfriend, Buster Bill Harris. Buster worked for a secondhand car dealership, and would sometimes show up on Friday nights, often in a sporty MG sports car he was trying to sell. I would wake to his snores on Saturday mornings from the mattress under the window of my small bedroom next to Mummy's. I never found out if he started out the night in her bed, but I like to think so. He would give me a shiny shilling to run to the newsagent down the hill for the *News of the World* (for the scandals) and the *Daily Express* (for the Giles cartoon and the racing form). There would always be enough left over to throw in the *Dandy* and *Beano* comics for me.

Buster was the closest male figure I had throughout my boyhood. I can still see the sleek line of his military moustache, the gleam of his bald pate encircled by an arc of Brylcreemed black hair, can still sense the aroma of his Prince Albert Crimp Cut pipe tobacco, the gleaming polish of his two-tone shoes, and most of all the rippling power of his brawny forearms. When I was still small enough to cuddle in his lap, he would swing his legs apart without warning, so that I would tumble perilously towards the floorboards, only to be grasped securely then promptly scolded for not sitting still. I never tired of this game and bless his heart, I don't think he did either.

As I grew older, the two of us would take off to watch the Saturday afternoon rugby games at the local club ground. Buster had a peaked tartan cap and a shooting stick; you pushed the pointed end into the earth and the top folded out to form a narrow leather seat to perch on. I've never seen another one since. Mostly though, we would tramp up and down the touchline to try to keep warm on those blustery winter days as he brushed me up on the finer points of the game.

Grandma heartily disapproved of Buster and whatever intimacy may have existed between him and Mummy. If someone in the family spotted Grandma heading across Bristol Road towards our house, it was my job to help Buster roll the telly—which we had rented for the weekend of Queen Elizabeth's wedding and somehow never cancelled—into the pantry, where he and the telly would hide out together till she left. One Friday evening he showed up with a rare breed of puppy, a Duke of Beaufort kennel terrier, and my sister Jane and I were led to believe he was ours to keep. Or maybe we just chose to think so. He was a tough and tireless black-and-white short hair, and it was a joy to watch him tear across Weston sands, chasing every other dog within view clear off the beach.

We christened him Spike, and it was Spike who introduced me to sex: early one morning he came romping through the kitchen door after escaping through the back gate. His proud penis was still erect and dripping. Jane and I were heartbroken when he had to go back to his Bedfordshire kennels for stud purposes, but I expect Spike got over the loss pretty quickly. Then one day came the equally unheralded disappearance of Buster himself. He had become *persona non grata* with Mummy as well as with Grandma, and there were no more weekend visits. But I wouldn't trade all my heartaches for those many male times he and I spent together.

Growing up with three older sisters never did unravel the shadowy mysteries of womanhood for me. Elizabeth and Mary, "the big ones," were for all the world grown-ups, while Jane and I, "the little ones," were at least for a few precious years playmates. We would share the same bathtub and snuggle together under the blankets on winter nights, or in the deliciously warm laundry cupboard during games of Sardines (an English version of Hide and Go Seek).

The two of us took several holidays to Devon together after we had left our early childhood home, staying with one of the farming families Mummy must have kept in touch with from earlier days. We got to join the farm workers in the fields for delicious Devonshire teas, then would sit on the back of the hay wagon wending its way down narrow winding lanes back to the farm. We would let our legs dangle down as we watched for the next fresh horse turds to plop down steaming under our feet. Jane would always rush to my rescue when one of the kitchen maids started bullying me. And she was a skilled mentor in teaching me the art of mud pie making, watching out that I didn't fall into the stream while I leant down to drink from it. It smelt and tasted of ferns and a little of cow dung.

Elizabeth was the academic in the family, always hidden away in her bedroom cramming over her homework. But I do remember more than once bursting in on her accidentally on purpose as she sat close to her boyfriend Peter on the drawing room sofa. Mary was the tease, and the only one not in the least bit scared of our father while he was still around. As a young child, she would sometimes bang on everyone's door early in the morning, shouting in her pronounced lisp, "Get up, you buggers, get up, you buggers!" (a very bad word in England at that time). Mary and I were the two early risers in the family, and once we caught a rabbit in the fields and hung it by its hind feet in the larder for several days. When we finally set about skinning and preparing to dress it for the stew pot, it took us only a few rank moments to realize our attentions were well overdue: putrefaction had set in.

St Peter's, which I attended from aged seven to twelve, was a private school with high fees, but thanks to a means test, Mummy never had to pay a penny for my education. I sensed, without ever being directly told, that non-private schoolboys were off limits as friends, but we dayboys at St. Peter's learned in turn the subtle lesson that we were lower on the social scale than the boarders. English class distinctions are largely unspoken but they run deep, something less apparent in North America. Classism is one of the most insidious and pervasive of social oppressions and of course hurts us all. Nowadays I like to remember that I am absolutely of the working class. It happens that I work very much with my head, but I've always worked with my hands, too. My whole childhood, though, was spent satisfying adults who fussed at me that I must "get ahead." My Aunt Ella, Mummy's cousin to whom I grew close after Mummy's death, would often remind me that I had a "first class brain," as though my whole future depended on my getting top marks in our pernicious grading system. How much healthier our society would be if we could dismantle these degrading class distinctions between us.

In September and October, as we dayboys made our way down Bristol Road to St Peter's, we would drag our feet through the leaf mounds to kick free the sweet chestnuts and conkers (horse chestnuts) that had fallen from the overarching trees. Budding capitalists that we were, we would exchange the sweet chestnuts inside their prickly green cases with the boarders for barley sugars, or even peppermint creams—one nut, one sweet in exchange. The horse chestnuts had a quite different purpose—the traditional game of Conkers. We would drive a skewer through the core of our chosen "cheggie," string it up on a sturdy stretch of string—often a shoelace—and tie a couple of knots at the bottom so it wouldn't drop through. Then we would pair up with an opponent and take it in turns to swing our conker at the other's stationary one, trying to smash it to bits. In the unlikely event that our newly-strung conker (called a *one-er*) cracked a gnarled and scarred victor of perhaps ninety-five battles (a *ninety-fiver*), our brand new specimen would at once be promoted to the status of a *ninety-sixer*. It would then be subjected to repeated challenges until it too flew and fell to a glorious death among the littered shells and thin patch of grass beneath the chestnut trees.

There were some time-honoured elements to the game. Hardness was the whole point—the harder the better. Be sure the surface of any newly selected specimen is smooth, because chipped ones split too quickly. Don't take on boys with cheggies that have survived many skirmishes until you have worked your way up through the ranks of five-ers and ten-ers, picking up a few toughening scars on the way up. And practice that swing—don't waste a whole turn with a total miss. Last but by no means least, beware heaped autumn leaves in the woods—all too often one of us would be fiercely stung after plunging an eager hand into a well-concealed wasps' nest.

Every one of the ninety-eight boys at St Peter's wore an identical uniform of grey caps, suits with short trousers, and knee-high socks. A band of royal blue encircled both caps and sock tops and ran diagonally down our ties. We were in trouble if we were caught outside any building with our caps *off*—or inside any building with them *on*. There developed a kind of liminal doffing and donning ritual at any school entrance: a peculiarly senseless rule that we broke whenever we could get away with it. We dayboys always seemed to be more scruffily dressed than the boarders—missing a jacket button or one of the elastic bands that held our socks up, so they drooped at half-mast. There would be mud on our grazed shins or damp grass on the seat of our trousers from rolling downhill in the park near the school.

We entered the school gates every morning as a defiantly united gang. The many daily games we played together taught us to be good sports, get along, solve our own problems, and stick up for ourselves. We had our rivalries, our tiffs, even occasional full-on fights, but they never lasted long. We were numerically in the minority by far from the boarders and separated by an invisible wall of money and class. Several of us were on scholarships, while the boarders' parents all paid the substantial tuition fees. If we rarely fought among ourselves, we often found occasions for not-so-friendly skirmishes with rival gangs of those toffee-nosed boarders we considered tough enough to earn our attention. We in turn learned to look down on the boys who went to the County Council schools and wore no uniforms. It would have been unthinkable to befriend them, though sometimes we got into scuffles on the way home from school, because for these working-class boys a cap from one of us who went to the nobs' school was a prized trophy.

In the spring and summer, Mummy would often be out in the garden planting out annual flowers, peas and tomatoes, or just cleaning up the winter's debris. I would sometimes come home from school to find her almost in the same place, as though she hadn't been back inside all day. She often used to tell us four children to "listen to the flowers"—we would probably call her a plant whisperer today. I was a mummy's boy until I went to St Peter's, so as a single parent she set about toughening me up. I remember she stopped hugging or kissing me once I turned six. Then in my first term at St. Peter's I was pushed in terror into the boxing ring for the first round of the house matches.

To my astonishment, I found in myself an angry little fighter who delighted in bloodying noses, even those of my friends. I can still feel that frisson of excitement when I would bunch my seven-year-old fists into those scarred school-issue brown gloves. The boxing master, Captain Lancaster (Capio), tugged hard on the laces to knot them tight about my wrists. Then came the queasiness in the pit of my stomach as I awaited my turn to duck between the ropes, step out onto the canvas with its smell of stale sweat and sawdust, and turn to blue or red corner, avoiding all eye contact with the boy a hundred miles away in the opposite corner.

With the strident command of the bell to commence the first round, everything vanished from my awareness except the savage joy of fists pumping into my opponent's face, the almost equal exhilaration of getting caught myself, seeing stars but utterly oblivious to my shredded lower lip. I would quickly abandon the strict boxing instruction that Capio had taught me: "Left arm and foot forward in a side-on stance, right hand up close to guard your chin, elbows together to protect your midriff, circle to the right watching for openings." I would simply rush in swinging, rarely ducking to avoid a blow, going at the boy right opposite without let-up while the world stood still around me.

I don't know where all this violent pent-up energy came from, but I must have been an angry child. Looking back over my forty-plus years of avowed Quaker pacifism, and of striving for loving kindness toward the countless children and families who have come under my care, I sometimes wonder if it's the same heart beating in me today as the one I was born with. My schoolmasters, and perhaps even Mummy, might have claimed that this bravado that carried me defiantly through so many boxing matches, as well as many bouts of corporal punishment as a teenager at boarding school, helped form my character. I don't think so. There are better ways to channel a child's aggressive instincts. Boys and girls are more self-confident and emotionally stronger who have had consistently loving relationships with the adults around them, rather than being urged into aggressive competitiveness from early on in life. Let alone told to have a stiff upper lip in the face of adversity and pain.

Learning from Disaster

The downhill tramp, the stripping naked on winter stoops,
the lye soap on cuts, scrapes, inky grunge: I never saw one flinch

"They always die at night?" I queried my uncle as we climbed the back stairs past a pungent midden.

"Pretty much. They seem to wait till dark."

I was on yet another house call in the early-morning hours with Uncle Ken, the sole doctor for three thousand miners and their families in this hub of Britain's coalmining industry. A flu epidemic had swept the West Riding of Yorkshire this Christmas season, and the mine workers, their lungs already coated with coal dust, had no defense against this devastating infection. They were dying like flies.

After our mother's death, my sister Jane and I had made the journey from the south to the north of England to live with my uncle and aunt during our holidays, though we had both stayed on at our high schools down south. The alien dialects that beset us on our train journey north left us with a schizophrenic sense of living on both sides of the ancient north-south divide—belonging neither here nor there.

My night vigils with my uncle over these exhausted men became a ritual whenever I was home from Epsom College, my boys-only boarding school in Surrey's stockbroker belt. I was well aware of Uncle's purpose—to cure me of my idiotic resolve to go to medical school. But it had quite the opposite effect. Not only did I find the families grateful to have a listening ear for their stoical tales of woe, but something often sprung free in my uncle, too. He had always been a storyteller and, having nothing else to offer but his bedside presence, he seemed to take some comfort from memories of other visits, and the intimacies that had grown up over the years.

“Most of them I delivered, too. Cradle to grave I’ve known this one,” he would tell me. “Breech delivery, he was. Got a scar under there from the forceps.”

“Was that at night, too?”

“Yes. Midder’s mostly night work. And they’re almost always born at home. I hardly send a one to the Infirmary. Tough, these womenfolk. They’ll labour fifteen, twenty hours before they even call me. They keep the pub open for the men. The grandmas deliver more than a few—often have the placenta waiting for me when I get to the house, just to check it’s intact.”

He recalled his first week of practice, the pithead bell peeling the end of the day shift, the tramp-tramp-tramp of coal-black men. An army marching down the steep cobbles, wheeling off one-by-one at each front door. “They strip naked on the stoop, all weathers, scrub off the coal dust in a basin of icy water and lye soap the wives leave on the stoop out front. They’ll not let them inside till they’re spotless.”

We were back at another bedside later that week. Though the man was barely forty, to me he looked seventy. I thought at first he was dead, his breathing so shallow in the gloom I could hardly detect any movement of his chest. I tuned into the short, sharp talk between wife and uncle, struggled to decipher it.

“Reet sorry to bother ’ee, Doctor.”

“How long’s he been like this?”

“Bin flaggin’ a week, like. Liggin’ int’ bed sin’ t’ weekend.’

“Why didn’t you call me sooner?”

She looked embarrassed. “’E tol’ me not to, Doctor.”

Uncle sighed, stifled a yawn, pulled out his ancient stethoscope from its accustomed place in his worn black bag.

“Maybe earlier we could have done something, Elsie.”

She flinched. “Aye, right gormless I were, ’arkin’ to ’im.”

Uncle looked chastened. “It’s no bother, you know.”

“’E said ’ow thee can’t kwacken a dyin’ man, Doctor.”

These stark intimacies—between miner and wife, wife and uncle, uncle and me—stoked my flame and sealed my fate. Robbed of witnessing my mother’s death, her cremation, or even her memorial service, I was granted a place of privilege at these thresholds. At these life-to-death transitions of Yorkshiremen distant from me in class and know-how as any on our island. Instinct guided me to forge brief links with the wives, even the children who would hold their own nocturnal vigil beside me. I started to grasp something of their vernacular.

“Canna get ’ee summat to sup, lad?” an elder daughter quizzed me. A girl-woman of seventeen, her beauty masked by fatigue.

“No, no, I’m fine. Please don’t trouble.”

“Nay bother, lad. Bah gum, thee looks jiggered. An’ famished.”

“Well, perhaps a cup of tea, then.”

“I’ll go mash the pot. Cut thee and ooncle some slabs of Parkin wi’ it.”

I blinked back unmanly tears at her kindness. *No blutherin’ at this bedside.*

Uncle’s stories continued. Lessons in awareness, witness, toughest love. Lessons to last. But traveling throughout my teenage years, between the upper-middle-class southeast of England of my boys-only boarding school, and the deeply industrial working-class West Riding of Yorkshire for my holidays, I never got over that ancient north-south divide that dates back at least to the Norman conquest. As a diffident teenager, I was acutely aware of my BBC accent, which the Oxford English Dictionary still defines as “the standard accent of English spoken in the south of England.” In the past it was termed *The King’s English*, or even *Public School Pronunciation* (the term public school having long been associated with independent fee-paying boarding schools, as opposed to non-fee-paying state schools. Go figure).

I knew only too well, without ever being explicitly told, that such an accent was associated with undeserved power and privilege, and that it had a strong link to the ruling class and British nobility. Nancy Mitford and others took things a step further by separating the English language into *U* and *non-U*, to distinguish upper-class from lower-class speech. The words *napkin, sofa, lavatory*, and *pudding* were all okay U-words, but God forbid you get caught using the non-U *serviette, couch, toilet*, or *sweet*.

It didn't help to be saddled with a double-barreled surname, which seems to have been in my family since a John Pole married a Rosina Graham several generations back. I had always assumed they were died-in-the-wool Southerners, but Sarah my niece, who has made a study of our family genealogy, just found out that John and Rosina hailed from the Shetland Islands—about as far north in the British Isles that you can get. But this practice of double-barreled naming originated with the British aristocracy, for whom wealth and prestige have always been major factors in negotiating marriages. While I made a few friends during my holidays in Yorkshire, I never met anyone who laid claim to a double-barreled surname, or talked with my BBC accent, or went to a fee-paying school. Among my teenage acquaintances, the *h* at the beginning of a word would always be dropped, and the *g* at the end of a word would never be pronounced. *The* and *to* were simply *t*, and anything and nothing were always *owt* and *nowt*.

But after a few pathetic efforts, I soon realized any attempts to merge in by adopting a Yorkshire accent was doomed to embarrassing failure. Thanks to Uncle Ken, I finally caught onto a few words of pure dialect: *liggin* for lying (in bed), *blutherin* for crying, *brass* for money, *gaffer* for boss, *reet* for right, *od thi' osses* for hold on a minute, and *tarra* for goodbye.

The whole time I lived in Yorkshire, Uncle Ken and Auntie Joan never left the county to journey south. Summer always meant a two-week car journey to the small seaside resort of Sandsend on the North Yorkshire coast. My uncle was a desperately nervous driver, and I was assigned to sit upfront as navigator, while Auntie Joan and their three daughters crowded into the back of his ancient Ford

Popular. No one had spotted I was growing increasingly short-sighted and could barely read the names of the multitude of narrow streets as my uncle negotiated his way through the dense township of York. Being the only one allowed to open his mouth, he did so to yell frequently at me for getting us lost under the battlement walls of the ancient city.

The culmination of the war between our two egos came in my sixteenth year. It started as a one-sided rant in the sitting room after Auntie Joan and the girls had all retired to bed. I was stretched out on the sofa, one eye on the TV and the other on Uncle Ken. He was standing over me bellowing once more about the cost of seven years at a London medical school—quite out of reach for an overworked and underpaid GP. I had never before found words to counter him, but a voice deep within me suddenly screamed *Enough!* I swung my legs down and stood up to face my uncle, no more than a foot of space between us. He was all too aware of my prowess in Epsom College's boxing ring—and it was at once apparent to us both that my recent growth spurt had given me both height and reach advantage.

"Don't ever yell at me again! I don't need any help from you!"

The words came out with the force of a right hook to his jaw. But my intense urge to lash out with both bunched fists was almost instantly disarmed. Uncle's look of stunned alarm had given way to something akin to awe. His next words almost caused me to fall back onto the sofa.

"John, I'm proud of you! Thank you for standing up to me!"

Hard to come up with a more literal description of my actions. After only a brief pause my uncle went next door to the kitchen and reappeared with two bottles of Tetley's Bitter. We christened this unlikely start to our newfound friendship with my first taste of Yorkshire ale. Healing takes many forms.

Ten years on, I would recall those moments as we shared more bottles of beer. I had taken time out from my medical internship at Barts to sit once more in Uncle Ken's sitting room. Two doctors exchanging stories, talking shop: the one callow but passionate, the other shortly to find his career of unremitting toil coming to an abrupt end with the onset of oesophageal cancer. The healing between us continued over several more visits in his final weeks. I'd long forgiven this man who had waited three full days after Mummy's death to summon me home as a first year boarder at Epsom to announce with no preamble or semblance of empathy that she was dead. With hindsight I came to know it wasn't in this repressed man to comfort me or to openly share his own grief at the loss of his beloved sister at fifty-one.

Back at Epsom for the summer term, I got an unexpected letter from Mummy's cousin, my Aunt Ella. I remembered her a little from visits as a young child to South Wales, but we had had no contact in recent years.

"John, Uncle Roger and I want to come to Epsom for Founders' Day," she announced. Founders' Day was my school's annual celebration, when parents were entertained to tea in a massive marquee erected in front of the college, and the First XI cricket team took on their closest rivals—usually St. John's, Leatherhead, or Charterhouse. Aunt Ella and Uncle Roger duly arrived, and he and I sat in front of the pavilion watching the game in silence but with mutual enjoyment. My only discomfort was hearing Aunt Ella's frequent shrieks of laughter from the tea tent where she was busy making the rounds of masters and parents.

They became faithful visitors after that, and I gradually stifled my embarrassment at Auntie's gregarious behavior as she introduced herself to all and sundry, while Uncle Roger held back—as taciturn as she was voluble. I took to visiting them twice a term for *exeats*, catching the train on Friday afternoon from Epsom Downs station up to Paddington, then the tube to Oxford Circus to meet her at the TB Clinic where she was head nurse. By that time—the late 1950s—there were several effective drugs to treat tuberculosis, but there were still occasional outbreaks, especially in southeast London where poor housing and overcrowding were still prevalent. Aunt Ella was often kept busy well into Friday evening, and I'd make myself comfy in one of the unused offices, where Flo the tea lady would keep me supplied with sticky buns and "a nice cup of char."

At last, Auntie would be ready to take off around the corner to Sherriffs wine bar, where I was introduced to the delights of Harvey's Amontillado sherry. My penance was to have to run the gauntlet of her friends and—for all I knew—perfect strangers with whom she had struck up acquaintance. Finally, we would be off to Liverpool Street station toting countless bags of groceries from nearby Berwick Street market in Soho, where fruit merchants and fishmongers have been plying their trade since the eighteenth century. Uncle Roger would meet us at Billericay station, the commuter town where they lived twenty-five miles east of the city of London.

I got to know a good number of young men during my visits to Billericay, and soon after I passed my driving license after four tries we had a memorable holiday on the Costa Brava. Eight of us travelled in four cars—two E-type Jaguars and two Mini Coopers—via the ferry from Dover to Calais, racing each other southwest across France and over the Pyrenees mountain range. We stayed in the small coastal village of Calaela de Palafrugell east of Barcelona in a flat above a small bar, where a bottle of Spanish champagne cost the equivalent of a dollar.

We would sleep off our hangovers until lunchtime, when our Spanish hostess and cook would rouse us with a magnificent lunch. After toasting ourselves on the beach all afternoon, we would play cards until it was time to head out for the Barcelona night spots. I taught the rest of them *Donkey*, a simple but uproarious card game with one house rule: whoever became the donkey at the end of each game headed downstairs to replenish the champagne supply. For reasons I never discovered, though I strongly suspected a conspiracy, I became Donkey at least ninety percent of the time. Maybe I just couldn't hold my booze as well as my buddies.

Early in my second-year internship at Barts, Aunt Ella and Uncle Roger retired back to South Wales where they both had family. But their retirements were short lived. First, Uncle Roger had a massive stroke which left him unable to speak, though he made more effort to do so after this tragedy than he ever had done when he was still totally healthy. Then Aunt Ella developed an inoperable cancer, just like my mother. She lingered on for many weeks in a comatose state, probably caused by both the spread of the cancer to her brain and the regular opioid medication she was receiving.

I couldn't get away from my job for several weeks, but finally drove the 150 miles from my Tufnell Park flat in north London to Cardiff General Hospital. The staff nurse directed me to a private room where Aunt Ella was lying mute and immobile—such contrast to her usual joyful volubility. She was seemingly quite unaware of my presence, breathing only periodically with an intake of breath followed by no breath at all for several seconds before there would be another gasp. This pattern was something I'd learned to call Cheyne-Stokes breathing—an ominous feature of someone not long for this world.

I pulled up a chair beside her, grasped her hand, and spoke quietly to her.

"Hallo, Auntie. It's John. Sorry I couldn't get here before."

As I watched, she let out one more breath, which proved to be her last one on Earth. It felt as if she had been waiting for me.

Scene of a Battle

sans ring, sans gloves, sans judge, sans rules:
a bare-knuckle prize fight with a bloody prize

I went to Barts Medical School in 1960 on an arts scholarship, meaning I had spent my last three high-school years studying exclusively the classics and history. I had to somehow cram two years worth of physics, chemistry, and biology into my unwilling skull in my freshman college year, acquainting myself in depth with something for which my mind had zero inclination. But somehow it had to be done if I was to fulfill the dream born in me at twelve years old with my mother's death. Somehow, I scraped through.

Once my second year was underway and I was introduced to anatomy, physiology, and biochemistry, I began to sense some kind of link to my chosen career. But by now I was also in the habit of hitting the pubs and savouring the countless other diversions London had to offer. I swiftly abandoned what had been for the past year a nightly routine of poring over textbooks, assigning that task to the week before each exam rolled around. I would then knuckle down to frantic all-nighters in the hope that I would hang onto enough information to scrape a pass and move on.

I had moved out of my comfy digs in Tulse Hill in South London into a flat with my new friend, Barry Goldhill. My primary motivation was my landlady's concern that I was getting far too friendly with her daughter, a first-year physiotherapy student at Brunel College. That, coupled with the fact that the last buses to Tulse Hill left central London at 11 o'clock at night—an hour when the student parties were just getting into full swing. I had become close buddies with Barry during my first year, perhaps seeing him as the older brother I had never had because he was two years my senior. He was also the only Jew in our medical school class, and

I felt drawn to him after becoming aware of the covert anti-Semitism prevailing among my other classmates. I am ashamed to remember betraying him more than once by smirking at ungentle gentile jokes at his expense, rather than standing up for him.

Barry and I moved into the fully furnished ground-floor flat of a 1930's house in North Finchley, owned by Mr. Peddici, a Greek Cypriot who ran a small greengrocery on nearby Archway Road. We made a point of faithfully buying his produce to offer penance for ruining his furniture and running late on our monthly rent. Arriving at a friend's party one Friday night after closing time at the pubs, we were disgruntled to find the usually eager nursing students had already fled to bed. On the journey home in my already battered primrose yellow Mini, a sturdy wooden roadblock partly impaired my progress. Several unidentifiable fragments detached themselves and accompanied us for the rest of the journey, clattering rhythmically against my front fender.

Once home, Barry proposed a bare-knuckle fist fight, I'm sure recalling brash boasts about my exploits as captain of the Epsom College boxing team. I teetered across the threadbare patch of grass that fronted our flat, chuckling about nothing in particular until Barry's left fist delivered itself of the weight of English anti-Semitic oppression directly onto the gentile nose of his best friend.

The ear, nose, and throat surgeon on call for Barts' Emergency Department doubled as associate dean of the medical school. My semiconscious state spared me from offering a detailed history of my current medical condition, which must have been plain enough to all present. I awoke several hours later with searing mid-facial pain and an awareness of a shield encasing my upper face like Duke William of Normandy's helmet. Was it then that the seeds of my later Quaker pacifism were sown?

I turned my head a cautious inch and dimly spied Barry sitting close beside my bed. It turned out he had not only got me to Emergency unaided but had stayed close by my bedside as soon as I had had my broken nose restored and was safely settled in a post-op bed. I was released the next morning, but not before the dean had delivered himself of an admonishing chat with us both about what Barts expected of its students. The soul of contrition, Barry made a point of accompanying me to my follow-up appointments and fending off inquiries from other students about the cause of my black-and-blue facial features.

Barry seemed to have connections in many quarters and was always finding us jobs that not only paid well but came with perks such as free drinks, or tickets to various performances. I was often invited to his home in East London, where his mother would serve delicious gefilte fish, brisket, potato latkes and of course delicious soup full of light and fluffy matzo ball dumplings. Back at the flat, I became by default the chief cook and bottle washer, unless we could prevail on one of Barry's seemingly endless succession of girlfriends to take over this role. Cooking was very much a trial-and-error experience for me, though it offered invaluable training for many future cooking experiments.

One of Barry's girlfriends, Lithuanian Rita, became a more permanent presence and finally moved in—three living cheaper than two. I would come upon them making love on the kitchen table, Barry observing the long-ordained rules of snooker by keeping one foot resting firmly on the floor while taking his shot. Rita was a gentile but Barry decided to make an honest woman of her despite the objections of his family. Early one morning the three of us took off to Finchley Road registry office, but were brought up short when the registrar inquired about the whereabouts of the second witness. Undeterred, Barry ran out into the street and persuaded a passing stranger to do the honours. Ten minutes later the loving pair had plighted their troth.

Barry never made it through our preclinical years, having failed every course exam at least once. But sometimes I'd take him to visit patients and he would find instant camaraderie with the many other Jewish East Londoners who made it onto our wards. After graduation, I lost touch with him, though I heard rumours he had joined his dad in his retail business. Five years later, I made it back to one of the regular Barts' reunion parties held in The Hand & Shears in Cloth Fair opposite Smithfield Market—the pub we students had always favoured. It was there that I learned that Barry was dead. He had driven his old blue Ford van, with its well-used mattress in the back, off the M1 motorway while heavily under the influence. I slipped away and shut myself in a toilet stall, where my tears flowed freely. In death, Barry had released the love I felt for him but had always suppressed while among my Protestant classmates. I saw him clearly as our sole Jew in the class, who had hidden behind a wall of defiance his bitter resentment towards the ill-disguised anti-Semitic world of postwar London.

Part Four

Play

Rock Star

I leaned closer and caught unmistakable fragments of "Lonely Hearts Club Band"

In my years at the University of Florida—from 1981 until my retirement in 2007—artful ways for healing became my primary focus as I committed myself to marrying art and science in my care of my patients. In the mid-eighties I embarked on what I have come to call my creative writing career, focusing at first on writing poems, then in 1991 nurse-painter Mary Rockwood Lane and I founded Arts in Medicine (https://artsinmedicine.ufhealth.org). We opened Shands Hospital doors to our first professional artists-in-residence very soon after, and in 1994 two members of the UF Dance faculty, Jill Sonke and Rusty Brandman, and I founded the UF Center for Arts in Medicine (https://arts.ufl.edu). Literally thousands of artists have given their time and talents to these two programs, but it has always been a special delight for me when a patient has shown an aptitude for expressing themselves in artful and creative ways.

Eli and Carl had been musicians from way back. When the brothers were fourteen and thirteen, they started their own rock band in their garage with three other school friends. Eli was the manager and Carl lead guitar and singer. At first, they reprised pop songs from past and present, but Carl showed a talent for composing and soon they had a growing selection of their own tunes. They did gigs at school dances around town and got a write-up in the local paper in their first season. Then Eli found himself slowing up, lacking his usual pizzazz. He would call a halt to rehearsals early, pleading schoolwork that he had to get done for the next morning. One evening when he hadn't appeared for an important rehearsal, Carl found him sacked out in bed.

"Hey Eli, what's up, man? We're waiting on you!"

"Gee, I'm sorry, guess I lost track of time."

Their mother at first put Eli's sluggishness down to burning the candle at both ends. She was used to having a hard time getting the boys moving on school mornings and she didn't think too much to it when Eli started missing out on breakfasts and barely making it to the school bus. It was only when he came home two days in a row complaining of a splitting headache that she took serious notice. She took one look at his flushed face and reached for the thermometer.

"We're off to see Dr. Phillips first thing in the morning, my boy," she told him, reading off a temperature of 101°. "Meanwhile, we're getting you to bed. But let's get some fluids and Tylenol into you first."

Eli didn't protest. When their pediatrician checked him out he found his glands were enlarged, both in his neck and under his arms, and he could feel the swelling of his spleen under the left side of his ribcage.

"Eli, I think you've got Infectious Mono—probably from all those girls you've been kissing. But just to be sure I want to run some blood tests. Your mom's prescription is right—rest, fluids, and Tylenol."

Two hours later, he called the boys' mother at home. "I've got those blood tests back. It's more serious than I thought. Eli's white cell count is sky-high. We need to get him in to see the hematologist at the university hospital today."

I saw Eli late that afternoon. Sure enough, his white count was in the hundreds of thousands, and I could see plenty of ugly looking cells when I looked down the microscope at his blood smear.

"We need to do a bone marrow test to find out more," I told him and his mom. Eli was looking relaxed if a bit flushed. "I think there may be something else going on. Examining your bone marrow will tell us for sure. Meanwhile, I think the best thing is to keep you in overnight."

Our first look at the bone marrow slides the next morning confirmed my fears. Eli had leukemia. Further tests told us it was of the myeloblastic variety, and he would need more intensive treatment than we use for the more usual lymphoblastic form of childhood leukemia. When I made rounds that evening, Carl was at Eli's bedside, together with both their parents. He had his guitar with him, and the boys seemed to be working up a new piece. Eli lay back on the pillows with his eyes closed, humming as Carl plucked the chords.

"Looks like they're getting ready to hang your chemo, Eli," I said. "We have to give you a bunch of fluids, so you'll be peeing like a racehorse. And we'll make sure you get plenty of anti-sickness meds. Tomorrow we'll get that IV port into you that I told you about."

I had gone over the protocol of treatment with the whole family earlier in the day. They all seemed to know just how bad things could be, the risk not only of the cancer but of its treatment. Eli's kind of leukemia requires high doses of chemotherapy to get the bone marrow into a state of remission; meanwhile there's a risk of serious complications—especially infections of every kind. And for reasons unknown, adolescent boys don't seem to respond as well as either girls or younger children. His parents asked all the right anxious questions; Eli meanwhile rested back in bed, mostly with his eyes closed.

"I guess we'd better cancel Saturday night's gig," he commented towards the end, as his father was signing the consent form for treatment to get started.

Things seemed to be going fine the first few days. Eli's temperature came down to normal, and the chemotherapy quickly chased his leukemia cells out of his bloodstream. We were starting to make rounds on the fifth morning of Eli's planned ten-day course of therapy, when the senior resident called me in to see him.

"He's spiked a temp of one hundred and three, and he's very confused. Looks like sepsis, or worse."

Worse meant meningitis or a brain abscess, both potential dangers to Eli's life. "Get a CAT scan stat and make sure we've got an LP tray ready," I told the resident as I went off to search for Eli's parents.

The lumbar puncture confirmed our fears—his cerebrospinal fluid was full of bacteria, and there was a striking paucity of healthy white blood cells to counter this invasion of his brain. This was hardly surprising; our chemo had put paid to all his healthy blood cells for some time to come. We put the chemo infusion on hold, substituting a combination of powerful intravenous antibiotics. Eli was becoming less and less coherent, tossing in his bed and clutching at his forehead as though in pain. We added a small amount of morphine and Ativan to the IV, fearful that we could easily overdose him and throw him into a coma.

"We need to move him up to the Intensive Care Unit," I told his parents. "If we don't get on top of this infection quickly, his blood pressure and breathing may become a problem, and we'd need to take steps to support them." I paused. "Things are going to be touch and go. Eli just doesn't have much to fight this infection with right now."

They had an isolation room set aside for him in the pediatric ICU. It was eight o'clock at night, and it didn't look as if the family was going to stray far from Eli's bedside. He was calmer but no more alert and his breathing seemed irregular. A nurse hooked him up to the monitor that would check his vital signs from moment to moment—pulse, respirations, blood pressure, oxygen level. Carl settled himself on the far side of his elder brother's bed, his guitar propped up in the window. I checked in with the ICU staff, knowing that he was in the best hands for any further emergencies.

"They'll call me right away if anything else happens," I told his parents. "I'll be saying my prayers tonight. He's still strong—he can pull through this."

They knew as well as I that Eli was about as sick as he could get, and he still faced an uphill battle even if he came through his current ordeal. I headed in early the next morning to find Eli almost as I had left him, apparently sleeping peacefully. No extra beds were allowed in the ICU in case they blocked access to the patient, so Carl and his parents had to improvise by each pulling two chairs together. I glanced up at the monitor, noticed his respiration rate had fallen; he was breathing at about twelve breaths per minute—abnormally slow though still quite regular. And he was maintaining his oxygen flow to his lungs without any added help from a respirator.

"When did he last get any sedation?" I quizzed his nurse.

"He hasn't had any since midnight. He's been pretty much out of it since he got here. They've ordered another CAT scan to make sure nothing new is going on."

Eli stayed in coma for four days. The CAT scan showed nothing new, and another lumbar puncture told us most of the bacteria were gone. But there was no sign of healthy white cells either in his spinal fluid or his blood. My own hopes for his recovery were ebbing. He seemed to me to be awaiting life's flight from its earthly beat. His mother had never left his bedside. I began to wonder if Eli was lingering here until she could finally offer his spirit up.

The fourth day, as I neared his room, I came upon Carl and the other three band members apparently engaged in an impromptu rehearsal in the passageway outside Eli's room.

"They said we could play for him if we kept the volume down," Carl explained.

After dutifully washing their hands at the basin in the anteroom, the band members crowded in around the foot of Eli's bed: a guitar, a base, and Carl and the fourth member on vocals. I lingered to listen. After a couple of numbers I didn't recognize, the room was suddenly filled with a rendition of "Good Morning, Good Morning" that bore an uncanny resemblance to the original track on the Fab Four's Sergeant Pepper album. This was followed by Carl's rendition of the closing number from the album, "A Day in the Life." For a few minutes I was back in the Beatlemania of 1960s London and my medical school years.

I looked around to see several of the nurses had crowded in the doorway to listen in on this impromptu concert. Meanwhile Carl lay quiet; there was no flicker of change in his vital signs.

"Hey, just because he isn't applauding doesn't mean he's not appreciative, you know," I told the band members. "Even people under full anesthesia can hear music. And perhaps Eli will be wondering if you're looking around for new management."

Three hours later, I was at my desk in my office, unwrapping my lunchtime tuna and watercress sandwich. The phone rang; it was Eli's nurse.

"I thought you'd want to know. Eli opened his eyes a bit ago, asked his mother where he was."

The next day Eli was sitting propped up in bed, eyes closed, but humming what sounded like a familiar tune. I leaned in closer and caught the unmistakable fragments of "Lonely Hearts Club Band."

Marshmallows

Physicians of the Utmost Fame
Were called at once, but when they came
They answered, as they took their Fees,
"There is no Cure for this Disease"

Hilaire Belloc

There's a term for it. For the grief we caregivers suffer when we lose one of our patients. We have this term, professional grief—a phrase that in its dry detachment captures the all-too-rare acknowledgment of the unexpressed feelings of professional caregivers. We may or may not have been trained to support and comfort the immediate family of one who dies, but few of us are taught to deal with our own often confused feelings of sadness and helplessness.

For myself, I have sometimes had recourse to laughter as a remedy—for my own professional grief, at least—even in an intensive care setting. One busy Friday, Betsy the PICU nurse manager asked me into her office for a chat as I was wrapping up my rounds for the day. I was aware that tensions had been running high on the unit recently after a series of sad happenings. She and I were good buddies and it crossed my mind she might want to get something off her chest.

"I've called a meeting of all my nursing staff," she started in without preamble. "They'll be here in a few minutes. Can you maybe join us?"

"Why'd you pick on me?"

"Well, you're up here a lot," Betsy responded.

True enough. Pediatric oncologists spend a good bit of time on this floor—and things don't often go too well.

"You're a good bit older, too."

"It's that obvious, is it?"

"Oh, you're still a kid to me. But they don't know that."

Betsy was referring to the seven nurses who were about to descend on her office. We both giggled—she was in her late thirties, and I wouldn't see sixty again.

"Well, I guess I've been around the block a few times. And I've probably got twenty years on any of our ICU docs."

"I haven't invited them, by the way. Just the nurses and you. They'll think you're here because of Ella."

Ella had been a patient of mine with a glioblastoma—an almost universally fatal brain cancer—and the most recent child to die on the unit. She had lapsed into a coma before she got transferred up from the pediatric oncology ward. If I'd had my druthers, I would never have moved her, but I've learned what hills to die on. The little girl hadn't been feeling much of anything when they put out yet another emergency call after she took her final breath.

"They don't have to know you're really here just to hold my hand if the going gets rough," Betsy added. "We've lost five patients in the past two weeks."

I knew what she was getting at. A couple of the senior nurses could be hard to handle. She'd called this meeting because of the tensions building between the nurses and ICU doctors. Rose—the nurse caring for Ella when she died—had come close to boiling point with the attending doc and his over-heroic efforts. Her opinion, anyway.

A brief knock on the door and the nurses began filing in. There were only two vacant chairs, so the rest sat on the carpet and leant up against the legs of the ones in the chairs. There was some friendly jostling as the room filled to capacity. I knew all seven nurses by sight, several by name. I sensed they all knew me—

the way nurses know all the docs who work on their unit. Things settled to an expectant silence, then Betsy looked around at everyone in turn.

"It's been real hard here lately, we all know that. So this is just a time and place for you to vent, share your feelings, anything you want."

Rose spoke right up. "Too right it's been hard. Some of those kids were never going to make it, Betsy. But the docs just can't seem to get it sometimes."

Annie picked it up. "Yeah, with that last code—as soon as Dave finally called a halt, he just went straight back on rounds. Like nothing had happened. Left it to the intern to break the news to the mom. Jeez, he's an unfeeling brute."

Her outburst gave everyone permission to blow the lid off.

"I never thought it could get this bad …"

"Five deaths in—what, a week and a half …"

"Some of those guys just don't know when to stop …"

"Maybe we should have called an ethics consult …"

"My boyfriend's getting pissed at me, crying every night …"

"Mine took off. I'm about ready to quit …"

The cacophony went on for several minutes. Two nurses were crying freely, feeling the unspoken permission, venting feelings too long held in check. A sense of release began to surface around the room, but Betsy let things run, knowing they needed to do this. As things quietened, she stretched out both hands to the two closest nurses, and the rest took the cue, hugging and holding hands. Tears gave way to brief grins. I laid a hand on the shoulder of Mia, whose back was propped against my knees. She freed her own hand, raised it to grasp mine and return my squeeze. My throat thickened. I grabbed at a handy box of tissues and blew my nose, then offered the used tissue to Mia. Grins became guffaws. Betsy took time to embrace everyone with her beaming smile.

“Thanks for coming—all of you. And feeling you could say your piece. We’ve all got a lot of crying to do. To hell with boyfriends who can’t hack it. There really are some good men out there!” More giggles. “Hey, maybe those attending docs could use a few hugs. Can’t hurt, might help!”

Rose looked at Betsy like she was about to nix the very idea, but she stayed quiet. Maybe even picturing the scene?

“Just be sure you don’t blame yourselves,” Betsy went on. “Like things could have turned out okay if you’d just done things a bit differently. Second-guessing can keep you awake all night.” She paused to take in everyone in turn. “Just know you did your best. I’m really happy you all decided to work here.”

Which got sniffles going around the room once more. I realized none of the nurses had launched any more attacks on the doctors after the first few salvos. The anger had surfaced fast and hard, then quickly opened up to expressions of grief. Like everyone knew it was the core thing, this big knot of helplessness and heartache. That shedding it was what this precious time was for—not for blaming absentee docs for their decisions and actions.

Rose freed up a hand to open a couple of packs of marshmallows. They made the rounds along with someone’s flask of Gatorade—no one seemed bothered about drinking from the same container. People grabbed handfuls like they hadn’t eaten for a week. Candy quickly started spilling. After a bunch of face-stuffing and munching, one suddenly flew through the air and caught Rose in the chest. Someone yelled, “Marshmallow fight!” cuing Rose to hurl several back in the general direction the first missile had been launched. Everyone began scrambling for larger handfuls and slinging them in random directions, tears giving way to screams and guffaws. After several minutes of bedlam, the energy started to stall.

Rose finally yelled out, “Okay, you can eat ’em all up now!”

There were no takers—most of the marshmallows had gathered a coating of rug or been ground under knees or butts. The brief feast over, we set about working with damp cloths from the bathroom, wiping off bits of goo from chairs and carpet.

"Anyone need their butt wiped?" Annie offered.

As I left, I checked my watch. Less than an hour—not too long out of a 168-hour week. And nobody was going to burn out today—someone's boyfriend might even get a big grin and a kiss tonight.

Pick up after Yourself

Eight-year-old Joey also found recourse to humour in a moment of tragedy. He had a horribly painful cancer in his hip that had shrugged off all our treatments. When mushroom balls showed up in his lungs it seemed almost merciful. His parents had been lying in wait when I emerged from Radiology after looking at those last hideous X-rays. As good a place as any to break the news, so I perched on the plastic chair next to Mom. She sat up straight and faced me full on.

"He's hasn't got long, has he?"

"No." I paused, holding her gaze. "A few weeks, maybe."

"Well, I want him to know fair and square, Doctor. We've never had any secrets in our family, and we're not about to start now. We want to make some memories, say goodbye properly." Her eyes flickered. "But we can't tell him. Can you do it?"

Telling an eight-year-old "fair and square" that he isn't long for this world is hardly an everyday task. But she was very clear—no ifs or buts. There weren't going to be any elephants in this family's kitchen. We gathered in my office: Joey, his parents, and me. "Square with him!" had been Joey's mom's last words. Her son looked out unblinking from his tucked-in-close place next to her on my beat-up couch. I felt the nakedness of his stare and knew I couldn't dissemble.

"Joey, you're going to die, go to Heaven."

My words were lost in an animal howl as he hurled himself into the recesses of Mom's yellow print dress. A big breath, then more sobs shook them both. The rest of us stayed silent, the collective grief threatening to swamp us. As Joey's keening gathered momentum, we eyed each other with the same unspoken thought: *Whatever else was right to do, this wasn't it.*

In reality, his howls lasted no more than a couple of minutes. Then on a long-drawn-in breath, his sobs ended as abruptly as they had begun. He swiveled his face out from his mom's arms, flicked a look at each of us in turn, spied our frozen faces. His gaze moved down to my office floor. It was littered with patient charts, medical journals, a bunch of photocopies, flotsam of a lunatic life. He looked me square in the eye.

"Didn't your mom teach you to pick up after yourself?"

It took the three of us adults a long moment to take it in—Joey had just come up with a *joke*. He had somehow decided in the midst of his distress that this would be a good time to lighten things up—for everyone's sake. With an eight-year-old's genius for putting strong feelings right out there, Joey had blown off his immediate fear and grief, then rapidly found space in his emotional toolbox for some healing humour. He had become in that moment the stand-up comic and thrown out this most apt of jokes.

He was grinning broadly, giving us permission to join him. Next thing, we were all down on our hands and knees giggling as we went about collective clean-up duty.

The Straight Poop

Twenty-year-old Natalie was one of the funniest, and pluckiest, patients I ever cared for. By the time she'd lived with her cancer for a year, she had found ways to talk to me out of earshot of her parents. She was in the habit of only bringing boyfriend Josh along with her to clinic visits, though she told me she kept her parents fully in the picture. I had my doubts, but I knew I couldn't call them up and talk behind her back.

She favoured a lively mix of jokiness and defiance, especially when it came to the tougher conversations. "Just the straight poop, okay? None of that flapdoodle you dish out to my folks." For a while now, the straight poop had been that her cancer was fast getting the better of her. The day I had to tell her what was in store in the near future, I went out to the waiting area to bring her and Josh back to an exam room—only to find the one vacant room I'd had my eye on was now taken. We stood around making small talk for several long minutes in the passageway—I wasn't about to launch into the heavy stuff in this bustling thoroughfare.

We finally got settled, Natalie leaning her full weight back against Josh on the exam table, trying to relieve the pain in her lumbar spine from the widespread cancer. I knew I couldn't dodge her demands for straight talk, but she took me right off the hook.

"I'm not scared of dying, Doc—I just don't want to do it in diapers!"

She threw a glance over her shoulder at Josh, who summoned a sheepish grin, though he was as near to tearing-up as I was. I had no answer to her levity, just a whopping lump in my throat. The odds were pretty short that she *would* end up in diapers.

"So you don't want to turn me into a guinea pig?" She was alluding to our earlier chat about alternative chemo drugs. She'd always let me know her dim view of *that* course of action.

"So—how long do I got?"

The way her cancer was spreading, she could be dead in a week. But Nat was some fighter. And if she decided she had things to get done, she might stick around for months.

"How long do *you* think you've got?"

"Hey, you're the doc, you tell me!"

Had I miscalculated by trying to toss in my own touch of levity, only to have it rebuffed? But her quirky grin told me I was in the clear.

"I wasn't really joking, Nat. People like you can have a lot of say about it. How long, I mean. You may have a few important things you want to get done before you go."

"Right! Like another weekend at Disney. So don't hold back on the morphine, Doc—I want to be able to make those rides."

Which at once took me right back to the day we had first met. It had been more than a year ago—the first Monday of the month, and I was just back on ward service. Nat had received her first heavy chemo course a few days earlier, and the mucous membranes in her mouth and throat were stripped raw. Mucositis is one of the worst and most painful of side effects from our chemotherapy. As I reached her bedside, she had grabbed a tight hold on my tie and rasped at me:

"Give me morphine!"

I made sure she got all the narcotics she needed as long as that awful pain persisted. Then three or four days later she had handed me a cartoon sketch showing an unmistakable likeness of her new doctor about to expire from anoxia.

The caricature of her own face was contorted like a four-year-old launched into a tantrum as she grasped my tie. Natalie had managed in that short time to look back on her recent terrible experience and summon up some quirky humour. This had pretty much set the tone for our doctor-patient relationship from then on in.

She was eying me steadily from the exam table. "It must suck having to tell people stuff like this. How d'you do it?"

Here she was with her childhood sweetheart, on the threshold of adult life, a young woman of brains and beauty with a newly awarded scholarship to the University of Chicago's graduate school. All to be cut abruptly short. Where did she find it in herself to offer *me* sympathy?

She went on: "That grad school money I've saved up—it'll help pay my funeral. It costs a bit, you know, getting buried. And Mom and Dad aren't exactly rolling in it."

She and Josh did make that last trip to Disney World, two twenty-year-old lovers who'd always insisted on being my friends—had never let "clinical" distance open up between us. Josh told me later that he'd made sure she was crammed full of morphine the whole weekend. But Nat was still with it enough to venture on several rides—putting a new twist on being high as a kite. Her man had been the one to change her diapers, though he never let on which bathroom they used.

"How are you holding up?" I asked him on the phone a couple of weeks after Natalie's death.

"Doing okay, Doc. About the last thing she told me was—I'd better treat any other girlfriends right, 'cos she'd be watching me from up there on her star. I believe it, too. I talk to her every night. She isn't far away."

My friend, Dr. Patch Adams, once challenged me, "Show me the data that solemnity ever cured anything." A lot has been written about laughter as a way of starting to heal from sad and painful situations, especially when we have no control over the reality surrounding us. Throughout my career as teacher, researcher, and caregiver I tried to marry art to science in healing—and to never overlook the art of humour. A teenage patient of mine once scolded me, "Lighten up, Doc—I don't need serious doctors around here!"—putting into words what many shyer patients may often have thought.

To Anatole Broyard, author of the memoir *Intoxicated by my Illness*, came "an irresistible desire to make jokes," when he found himself hooked simultaneously to IV and urinary catheters in his hospital bed. He cried out for "a witty doctor who could appreciate the comedy as well as the tragedy of my illness." Perhaps in his dying he recalled that mediaeval "death joke" played—wittingly or unwittingly—by Venetian plague doctors in the 1600's epidemic of *Yersinia Pestis—The Black Death*. Venice still found reason to celebrate its time-honoured public celebration—*lo carnevale Veneziano*. And like *commedia dell'arte* characters, those doctors donned bird-beaks full of dried flowers and spices to visit the sick. In these days of corona virus prevention, images of plague doctors are appearing on masks beside the caption, "Favorite Shopping Outfit."

Laughter can be an antidote to the isolation, dismay, even despair, we all feel in the face of overwhelmingly tragic events. To paraphrase G. K. Chesterton, children can fly because they take themselves lightly. Perhaps it's exactly because of their youth that so many patients I've known remained intensely alive almost until the moment they died. Perhaps we grown-ups can follow their example and make sure we die young as late as possible.

Ni Hao!

sheered-off cliffs close enough for old women to shake our hands as they broke from washing clothes in the junk-filthy water

I was talking to our friend, Cathy Lin, who works her magic to lift our HARP manuscripts (www.harppublishing.ca) off our computers and ready them for the printers. She came to Nova Scotia from China to study digital art at NSCAD University in Halifax, and our conversation put me in mind of the most exotic trip I ever made. I was among a group of physicians and psychologists who visited Chinese counterparts in 1990, the year after the Tiananmen Square massacre.

My first cultural awakening came on the almost 24-hour China Eastern flight between Seattle and Beijing. Recapturing my sleepless early-hours experience seemed to demand poetry.

East and West

I eye three hundred Asians: columns of forty, rows of eight,
cruisers on China Eastern's triple MD-11 turbofans heading
northwest from Seattle over Kodiak Island and the Arctic cap,
eleven-thousand kilometres across the dateline into the far east.

And notice each face is different, as I had always suspected.
Brittle-eyed at 4am US east coast time, I eye this cumulative
facial miracle, knowing we are ninety-nine percent identical,
but that one-percent represents such ineffable uniqueness
as to distinguish each of us from each other without thought.

As I sought out the washroom after checking into our Western-style Beijing hotel. I passed a tall silent elder standing stock-still in the doorway. When I came to wash my hands in the basin, I felt firm hands begin to caress my neck and shoulders, gently at first then with growing pressure. I looked up from my ablutions and our eyes met in the mirror. Neither of us changed expression as a brief vertical stroke down my upper back signaled the completion of my massage. I made a clumsy attempt at a bow, borrowing heavily from the movies. He bowed in his turn, bringing his hands up and together in the universal gesture of blessing. Our tour guide had already impressed on us—no tipping in China—but the urge to pull some of my newly acquired yuan from my wallet was hard to resist.

I woke at six next morning, pulled back the drapes and watched countless people performing *tai chi chuan* in their diminutive front yards. As we strolled in Ritan Park we saw large groups engaged in this same ritual, while an audience of old men hung their cages of canaries from the branches of the gingko trees. Walking four-abreast down the wide sidewalk back to our hotel, we collided with a man of seventy who strode backwards straight into us. He was understandably unused to huge Westerners spreading themselves across the pavement. After bowing in forgiveness-apology he resumed his steady march, still backwards, out into the six-million bicycle and tricycle throng on the street.

Trust

We decide the old man marching backwards
down the Beijing sidewalk is entranced: an effect
of early-morning tai chi chuan in Ritan Park.

So we four round him, resist trigger-happy snapshots,
move ahead, then stop abruptly at the crossroads,
leery, unlike him, that the bicycle tide will wash us away.

So he steps unpausing into the one on the left of our party,
beams on us forgiveness-apology, strides onward into the street.
We learn later he was simply strengthening his back.

The broad Guanghua sidewalk was scene to continuous colourful commerce. All kinds of strange produce from the surrounding countryside had been toppled from gunny sacks onto orderly lines of white sheets stretched out across the pavements. As we ambled along, taking in the gathering pace of the commercial activities, we learned another cultural lesson: the Chinese have no use for diapers.

Beijing Clean-up

Her small one squats in uncurbed glee on the busy sidewalk,
makes his deposit on the curb, awaits the newspaper
his mom is fetching from her tricycle at the curb.

Like an acrobat she twirls him face down on her lap
to wipe through the gaped triangle in his cut-out pantaloons,
then wraps the matter in the China Daily News.

They pass on unheeded together, he perched
in the carrier up front, she at her tricycle pedals,
weaving with seven million others along the spotless street.

We visited three of the city's largest hospitals, each boasting its own bone marrow transplant unit. Stem cell transplants are high-tech and extremely expensive in North America, but in China they were as low-tech as it gets. We watched a patient under a local anaesthetic of ten acupuncture needles having copious amounts of bone marrow removed from deep within his hip bones. It was reminiscent of NYT correspondent James Reston undergoing appendectomy under acupuncture during President Nixon's tour of China. But the most non-Western aspect of this current scene was the sight of a technician counting the bone marrow cells so far collected, using a microscope illuminated solely by daylight: the microscope was devoid of all electrical power.

We took a motorboat ride on the Gangiang Canal in Sujhou—known as the Venice of China, after Venetian traveler Marco Polo's visit in the twelfth century. A group of boys pursued us along the banks and over the bridges lined with crimson Chinese Firecrackers and white sycamore, calling out streams of "Hello, Hello!" to our echoing "Ni How's".

On the Ganjiang Canal

Venice has gondolas, Sujhou concrete barges:
they don't have enough *yuan* for the wood:
houses are set in the hull, tricycles in the bow.

Stone cottages—sheered-off cliffs—abut
enchanted junk-thick water. Once, twice, thrice,
our engine snarls in ginkgo leaves, plastic bags.

The rudder catches, knocks against a house door
as though demanding entrance. An old woman
washing cottons at her garden edge cackles at the scene.

She breaks off her ablutions to shake our hands
as backyard-onlookers and houseboat-people join the fun.
A gang of four chases us on crimson firecracker banks.

They call *Hello! Hello!* giggling madly at our echoing *Ni Hows!*
Then disappear elusive, pop up along miles of sycamore bridges.
Two speedboats splash us into Sujhou's Grand Canal.

The highlight of our stay awaited us at the 'Children's Palace' in the Xuhai district of Shanghai, which houses special after-school activities for gifted and promising children. There is a strong emphasis on artistic pursuits, and they had arranged a performance in honour of our visit.

China Childhood

The Children's Palace in the Xuhai district of Shanghai:
Our party is invited to the place of honour at the front
as five- and six-year-olds, some young as three, gather to perform.

Consummate soloists regale us on mystical *yan chin* dulcimer,
on two-stringed *erhu* and *pipa* classical guitar:
fifty short recitals conducted with serious formality;

there are no smiles or chatters or claps—such Western
ways to show appreciation. A brief pause in
respectful silence is the order of the day.

After two hours, the concert master takes her bow,
the children line up, silently bow in their turn. We bow back,
turn to the parents, bow to them. Still no word is spoken.

At an unseen signal, the three-to-six-year-olds become
children. They rush us *en masse*, mob us, eager to shake
Western hands, laugh madly, chase us up and down stairs;

a whirl of flying flower shirts, dungarees,
red, white and blue tights, spotless sneakers.
Ready for our own release, we enter into the fun.

We tear about the gym until no one knows who's chasing who.
The parents beam though none join in. Would I had been
a fly on the wall over Shanghai suppers that night.

The Actor

Four o'clock in the afternoon in the Child Psychiatry Unit: a low time for the group of teens assembled here. They were out of school and had time on their hands until supper—altogether too much time in this windowless room that served as second home to this gang of five teenage diabetics who wouldn't take their shots.

Each one of them knew full well what it meant, this non-compliance with their medical regimen. Diabetes is a killer, even in the young. Without the mandatory twice-a-day insulin shots, their blood sugar would run out of control, building up acids and other toxins in their blood, leading inexorably to shock, failing kidneys, and a coma from which there would be no waking up. Without the necessary medical intervention, that is.

This "necessary" intervention meant a lifetime stretching ahead of them of not only insulin shots but of strict control of everything they ate. It meant counting calories, it meant going without treats their healthy schoolmates took for granted. And even with strict adherence to their medicines and their lifestyles, there was no guarantee they would stay free of all the other complications diabetes lays on its sufferers as life goes along. Heart and circulation troubles, eye and kidney disease, and a horrible proneness to infections that are hard to treat.

These were smart young people. They had it figured out, and their normal teenage rebelliousness had turned against this act of God that had stuck them with a life sentence. It was as if they'd jointly decided—a life lived with diabetes just isn't worth it. A collective *why bother?* Which was how each of them had ended up here in Child Psychiatry. As far as their parents and their doctors were concerned, these children didn't have a choice. They were minors, after all, and each one of them had been indulging in enough at-risk behavior to cause them to get dangerously sick. Hence this spell in our child psych unit, separated from their healthy peers except on weekends, until they came around to accepting the hand life had dealt them. Compliance, or the lack of it, was the name of this game.

There was only one girl in the group. Linda was sixteen years old and had had diabetes for the last two of them. "It sucks, as far as I'm concerned," she told me. "I'm sick of all the rules and regs. I'm sick of the schedules. I'm sick of the shots. And all those yucky therapists, with their *analyzing*—they give me the creeps. I'm ready to do myself in some days, okay? So sue me, why don't you?"

My friend, Sid Homan, had been teaching medical students non-verbal communication for several semesters as part of our Arts in Medicine program. Sid was a professor of literature and theatre at our university, and a *tour de force* in the lively art of improv acting exercises. Now I'd invited him to start putting in weekly sessions with these diabetics, and here he was facing this gang of bored and resentful teenagers. Could he take them on—and could he win them over?

Sid took a long look around, rolled up his sleeves, stepped to the middle of the room, and took charge. "Okay! On your feet! Time to *act* like you're having a good time! Time to *play. Parts* I'm talking about!"

All five teens glanced briefly in his direction. He'd caught their attention despite themselves. *Who is this weirdo?* was the unspoken comment.

"Come on, it won't kill you. You don't have to tell me how fed up and miserable you are. I've seen lifers happier than you lot. Now off your duffs!"

One thing these young ones had learned here was that in the end it was easier to obey than to argue, even in goofy situations like the present. One by one they grudgingly hauled themselves to their feet and formed a ragged semicircle around Sid.

"Now, gentlemen, and lady"—with a theatrical bow toward Linda—"I'm going to teach you to *perform*—I mean, really strut your stuff! But first you've got to learn how to breathe with your bellies—like babies. Breathe *through* your bellies—so you can project your voices. Make yourself heard at any party!" This was all delivered in a parade ground bellow as he strutted up and down before the five of them, rubbing his hands red.

"Okay, let's try it. After three—'Abominable abdominals, abominable abdominals, abominable abdominals' … faster, faster … okay! Now—'Garlic gargle, gargle with garlic, garlic gargle, gargle with garlic …'" Then without a pause for breath he was into "'Lemon liniment, lemon liniment, lemon liniment …'"

Sid kept pouring on the tongue twisters at a faster and faster pace until the whole group was really *trying*. They didn't have time to ask themselves what the … were they getting into? The peer pressure kicked in among the four boys and they started trying to outdo each other. After a couple of minutes of facial mobility exercises ("How clowns like us warm up before going on stage," Sid told them), that gave them the chance to lay ghastly grimaces on each other, they were into "Bing, bang, bong, boppity, bop, bop, bop," a game that had them hopping and jumping as if their lives depended on it.

Only Linda was holding out. As the solitary girl she was acutely embarrassed, feeling suddenly vulnerable among the boys' snickering and jeering at each other's expense. A vulnerability she had managed to keep layered over pretty well in recent times. Sid quickly noticed how she was holding back and set about drawing her in.

"Okay, take a rest. You're good, you guys! You're getting into it." After a couple of minutes break: "Right, now I need a volunteer—preferably a girl. Let's see" (he made a big thing of looking all around the room)—"Ah! How about it—what's your name?" He was looking directly at Linda.

"Linda," she mumbled. She looked like she was struggling with the impulse to dash headlong from the room.

"All right, Linda. It won't hurt, I promise. I just need to see how you perform on stage. Ever been on the stage?"

She shook her head.

"Ever seen a live show?"

"Only on TV."

"Ah yes, but that's not *live.* I mean, when you're in the theatre, and the actors are real live people in front of you. Like you can see their make-up and so on. *That* kind of live."

"I guess not," she muttered.

"No mumbling now. I need *projection* if you're going to be an actor. You know what projection is, don't you? It's like being out on the street and talking to the farthest-away person in sight. So you want to be an actor?"

"Yeah, sure, cool." Linda had no idea where this was going, but she was not about to back down amidst this solidly male company.

"Okay, this is the deal. We're going to make up a dialogue, you and I. We're going to make like doctor and patient. Dialogue is what we call *chat* on stage. Only *you* get to play the doctor and *I* get to be the patient—sort of role reversal. Right, let's get some props."

Sid took a long look around before his eyes fastened on the boys ogling the scene unfolding before them.

"Hey, you guys, what're you standing around grinning at? Come on, see if you can rustle up Linda a white coat. Maybe a stethoscope. Must be one lying around here somewhere."

Two boys headed for the door. It seemed they knew exactly where to look. Inside three minutes they were back bearing their trophies. The doctor's white coat hung long on Linda, but the stethoscope they draped around her neck looked just the part. Suddenly she was a queen strutting among her courtiers. She grinned—she was getting into it.

Sid: “Alright, I come into your office, feeling sick as a dog. I’m looking for help. A little comfort. A little advice.” (Grimacing): “Hey Doc, I don’t feel so good.”

Linda (grasping both ends of her stethoscope): “Okay, so—where does it hurt?”

Everyone giggled. The idea of Linda playing the doctor was really getting to them.

Sid (making awful faces): “It hurts all over.”

Linda (light bulb going off): “Hmm—better get the shot box. Soon take care of that.”

Sid (hamming up the cringing and whining): “Oh no, Doc, not that, not the *shot box!*”

The banter swung back and forth, the two of them mostly standing toe-to-toe, like boxers fighting a battle of words and gestures. Magically, Sid had tapped into Linda’s own awareness of herself, getting her to break out of the fixed and crusted-over place she’d been stuck in, that no amount of psychotherapy had ever seemed likely to pierce. She paused for breath, tossed a look at the boys—a mix of defiance and pride. Gone was the self-pity and insolence, replaced by this colourful hamming up of her new role.

She eyed Sid. “This is cool, man.”

“Yup. You’re a natural at this role-playing stuff, Linda. So how are you doing?”

“I’m just getting it—this breathing through my belly.”

Rachel Triages

Rachel liked to spend her night times in the Emergency Room. Not as a patient though; she was an artist with a successful downtown studio. It's just that she found herself high as a kite after a twelve-hour spell at her canvases, and she had a hard time coming down and settling to sleep. Sometimes she could calm herself enough by creating funny collages. She kept a store of old magazines and delighted in thumbing through them till she happened on two images that made a jokey juxtaposition—the more absurd the better. She would glue two cut-out pictures on the same cardboard postcard—a boy in bathing trunks looking up from the bottom frame at the runaway railway engine in the upper frame passing right over his head. It seemed exactly as if nothing was keeping them apart.

But more often than not, shortly after midnight she would take herself off to our local community hospital emergency room less than a mile away from her studio home. Once she was in the waiting area she would set up her easel in one corner. There were always a few customers there, some of whom had been hanging out most of the evening waiting to be triaged for one of the night's overworked doctors to see. Triage is a word borrowed from battlefield parlance when a nurse has to make a quick assessment of each newly arriving patient, then decide who is most in need of the most urgent aid. Medicine is fond of borrowing war images to describe its routines.

For Rachel this was an ideal studio away from studio, given that the patients were often spending hours with nothing to help while away the time but desultory conversation with fellow sufferers and short naps in unyielding plastic seats. She picked out subjects to sketch who caught her eye; after all, this was what she did for a living. She'd never met anyone who objected, particularly when she donated her work to whoever she had picked out to sketch.

This particular early-early morning, Rachel was just setting up her easel in her accustomed corner when the door flew open and in burst a young man of maybe seventeen with unkempt clothes and eyes rolling like a maddened horse. He stared about him muttering, then started pacing the length and breadth of the waiting area, oblivious to the curious looks of other occupants. Up to this point, Rachel had been planning on sketching a collage of the family of four in the opposite corner, consisting of two bleary-eyed grown-ups and two school-aged children stretched out asleep head-to-toe on a bench. But the abrupt entrance of this young man at once diverted her attention. She watched him striding back and forth, asking herself if he was an addict looking for a fix. He didn't seem to be hurting physically, but he sure wasn't happy. Was he dangerous?

She eyed him for a few more moments, then selected a couple of brushes and assembled blobs of several different paints on her palette. She began to frame a preliminary sketch of the young man on her pristine canvas. She was intent on catching the agitation in each step, the to-and-fro twisting of his torso, the sudden swirl of his head. His contour began to jump out from under her brush as she moved to fill in her outline.

As he turned for the umpteenth time the boy stopped abruptly, at last aware of her focus upon him. As she glanced once more over the top of her easel Rachel realized she had made contact. She had definitely caught his attention. She wondered briefly if he was going to turn belligerent, but he simply looked directly at her before moving slowly in her direction. Although he showed no hint of threat, Rachel felt a flurry of nerves. She had never encountered anyone who had taken exception to her quiet daubings, but could this be a first? She grasped her brush tighter as though it were some kind of weapon that she could use to defend herself By now he'd drawn close and he came to a complete halt. He stood still for the first time since he'd entered the room. He was still breathing fast, and still had that bewildered look in his eye, but he was noticeably calmer.

Rachel slowed her own breathing as she let her eyes drop back down to her canvas, loosened her grip on her brush, and resumed work. When she looked up again the boy had drawn even closer. The wild stare had been replaced by curiosity. The scene became like a game she remembered playing as a young child. When she looked down at her work, he felt free to edge closer. But he was trying hard not to let her look up and catch him moving. He was now close enough to her canvas to see the beginnings of his portrait outlined in black, with as-yet-unformed daubs of colour within.

"That's me you're painting, isn't it?"

"That's right." She kept it nonchalant.

"What are you up to? I mean painting and all that?"

"I often come here. I like it. A lot of the folk I paint seem to like it too." She held his look, offered him a small smile. "Some people spend a lot of time waiting, so it gives them something to look at. I usually give them their portraits to take home if they want them."

He was silenced for a long moment, then, "I just came in here to get my meds. I have to take 'em, otherwise I get real anxious an' all." He was starting to display some of his earlier agitation. "The doctors say I mustn't stop taking 'em, but I ran out yesterday and I couldn't get hold of anyone in the doctor's office."

Now that he was close to her, Rachel took in the sweat on his cheeks and neck, and how his shabby tee shirt stuck to his chest.

"You mind me painting your picture?"

"No. No." He was getting self-conscious, making to smooth his hair straight.

"Better if you just relax. I don't want you posing for me! You can go on pacing if you want. Just take it easy."

"Okay. Cool."

He backed off a little, looked about him as if for approval and restarted his pacing—but with slower and more even strides. Every few turns he came back to gaze over Rachel's handiwork. The third time, he drew up sharp.

"Hey, that's really me. Yeah, you got it. Cool."

"You think? You like the look of it?"

"Yeah. Yeah. So you do this for a living, kind of?"

"Well, I don't make any money here in the ER! But yeah, I paint for a living."

"Wow!"

He was clearly blown away. Meeting a real live artist who made a living at it was too much to grasp.

"So what kind of pills are these you ran out of?"

"Oh, they're for my nerves. I get really upset and jittery without them. Like I said, I'm not s'posed to miss any or I'll end up in the hospital."

"Well, you seem to be doing pretty well right now. You think maybe you could last till morning? Doesn't look like things are moving too fast around here. But I'd love it if you'd stick around so I can finish your portrait. Then you can take it home with you."

"Yeah, okay. Hey, you know, maybe I don't need a doctor. I could just come back in here when I need to and get you to do another picture."

Part Five

Working the Front Lines

The Surgeon

On the telephone, amidst the unremitting noise of phones and typists, the bustle of staff scurrying between charts and patients, PC screens of appointments made, cancelled, and rescheduled, the clinic's receptionist could barely make out the words. The voice was as hoarse as a toad's, but much quieter. She recognized it at once for the esophageal rasp of one whose voice box was no longer working—or even present.

She had heard the like of it many times in her years in the Ear, Nose and Throat clinic. Try as she would, though, she couldn't detect the caller's name or whereabouts, let alone what he was calling about. But there seemed no nuance of urgency in the sounds. She handed the phone to a nurse who had come searching for a chart, to see what she could make of it. Whoever was on the phone seemed able to grasp instructions, so the nurse suggested he come on into clinic in the morning, so they could help with whatever was troubling him.

"We'll recognize him soon enough when we see him," she commented after hanging up.

I had known Keith for eighteen years. He was five when I inherited him from my predecessor. He was suffering from congenital laryngeal papillomatosis—a rare condition triggered by a viral infection acquired during pregnancy. Affected children develop warts—papillomata—during infancy or early childhood. These swollen purple monsters grow out from the upper air passages and in time can hamper the flow of oxygen. At first, they affect only the larynx but in bad cases they will stretch right down the bronchial tubes and deep into the lungs. If they really get going, they can become a big threat to breathing.

Keith was one of the rare and unlucky ones—so badly affected that all the drugs that work for others had never done a stitch of good for him. For the last dozen years, he had depended for his continuing life on a monthly surgical clearing of as many of these misbegotten giants as the ENT surgeon could get to. Quite early in his life, his voice box became so scarred that he had to have a permanent tracheotomy put in place, to bypass the larynx as a thoroughfare for oxygen to the lungs by opening a hole in the trachea below it. With a permanent tracheotomy, he had learned to make vocal sounds by using his gullet and could make himself understood well enough. But not when he was struggling for enough oxygen to stay conscious. And even in such a perilous state it was hard to put even a nuance of urgency into the sounds that came out of him.

He lived with his mother in a town of a couple of thousand people forty miles south of the university. He was largely confined to home, and at twenty-two he could take care of his medical needs when his mother went to her waitressing job at the local Denny's. There was only one way to keep the flow of oxygen into his lungs intact day and night, and at this he was adept. It called for suctioning—six, eight, even a dozen times a day—of his tracheotomy opening to drain the continuous build-up of mucus. This was the effect of the warts' permeating presence. It got a whole lot worse when the weather was cold: the build-up became much stickier and harder to adequately suction.

His mother had known for the past five years about Keith's greatest birthday and Christmas wish, although he had never mentioned it to her directly. It took her that long to put aside enough money to buy it for him: his own personal computer, together with a subscription to the Internet. Until then, his days had been solitary ones; he'd been home-schooled all his life, and few friends kept up with him. The Internet opened up a whole wide world of new acquaintances through the chat rooms and list serves that he joined. Some days he found himself getting flirtatious, though he knew it could never amount to more than an e-mail exchange of lighthearted endearments. But he was content enough with his sedentary life. And although the monthly surgeries left him raw and often coughing blood for days, he enjoyed the outings and visits with his nurses and doctors at the hospital.

But on this particular day, Keith was totally depleted of energy. He had felt under the weather when he went to bed the night before, knew he was coming down with a bug. This morning things were more of an effort than usual because his secretions were growing ever more tenacious. He hated his mother to fuss and knew only too well her need to put bread on the table for both of them. When she checked on him before heading out for her early shift, he stirred and muttered he was fine. She wasn't to worry about him—he was due in for his monthly clearing the day after tomorrow. He knew it would be none too soon, but he kept that thought to himself.

It was noon before Keith got himself out of bed to fix his breakfast. He liked to shave and look his best each day, even though he knew that most days the only people he would see were himself in the mirror and his mother that evening. As he peered at his reflection, he caught sight of something weird-looking in the area around his trach. As he leaned in closer the sight caused his heart to leap in his chest. No doubt about it—the tops of two polyps were protruding from the hole.

He had never in twenty years had a direct view of these turgid lumps, even though they had been his lifetime companions. Of their stealthy growth within his airway he had old acquaintance. He had often imagined them crowding and jostling like livid serpents along the walls of his bronchial narrows. Sometimes they would even invade his dreams, but they had never before taken living form before him. The sight of them poking their heads out into the world made him breathe even harder, forced him to struggle for each life-preserving gasp. It seemed futile to turn to the suction apparatus; that was only good for liquid secretions.

With a huge effort he made it to the telephone and dialed the number of the restaurant. One of the waitresses answered and recognized his voice at once.

"Your mom's on her lunch hour, Keith, said she was going grocery shopping afterwards. I'll be sure to let her know you called just as soon as she gets back."

It was then that he dialed the clinic, desperate to make himself understood and to summon help. He struggled to get a nuance of urgency into his voice, but the effort was too much. He was losing his remaining strength just trying to make himself understood to the two women on the end of the phone. He knew his access to oxygen was failing fast. When he heard Rita, a nurse he had chatted with countless times before, suggest he come into clinic in the morning, he gave up the effort.

It was then that he thought of it. He had been on the receiving end of the ENT surgeon's knife twelve times a year for more than a dozen years. He had surely learned something from these almost two-hundred surgeries. Had he not served an ample apprenticeship? He may not have access to his own operating theatre, but couldn't he still make shift? He thought about the knives in the kitchen drawer, then quickly decided the bathroom scissors would be easier and less risky to work with. He knew he must sterilize them as best he could, and that he would need a whole lot of something to mop up with. After hunting about in the kitchen and bathroom between longer and longer breaks to rest and catch his breath, he settled on two toilet rolls and a bowl of steaming hot water that he took the time to heat over the stove.

He set to work. Seating himself as close as he could get to the front of the bathroom mirror, he thanked his maker that his eyesight was strong. With a wad of toilet paper in his left hand, and his suction catheter close beside him to his right, Keith started snipping lightly at the swollen serpent heads protruding through the tracheal opening.

But he hadn't reckoned on just how bloody an operation it would quickly become. As the first scalp dropped to the counter, the blood started to spurt. After a desperate struggle, he finally succeeded in getting a grip on the remaining stalk that was sticking out of his trachea so that he could staunch the blood. With his other hand he directed the suction tube around his surgical field. Miraculously he was able to clear things enough to be able to catch his breath. After a couple of minutes, he cautiously released a little pressure from the site of his handiwork. He saw with satisfaction that the blood flow had almost ceased.

Time to snip some more.

Five minutes later his mother found Keith stretched out on the bathroom floor. He was still conscious, but there was a fast-spreading pool of blood around his neck and chest. When she had heard that he'd called, the instinct of a mother for her sick son at once asserted itself. She had known things didn't sound right that morning. Something bad had happened, she was sure of it. She had dialed an ambulance to meet her at the house before speeding home herself. The scissors and bloody toilet tissue lay on the counter. She figured out at once what he had been trying to do and cursed herself for leaving him alone.

Thirty minutes later they were in the hospital ER; thirty minutes after that he was in surgery. With even more than his customary painstaking dissection, the ENT surgeon was able to once more open up his airway. Keith came to in the Recovery Room to find his mother bending over him.

"Sorry, Mom," he rasped at her. "I thought I could do it."

She grinned tearfully. "Well, next time you decide on do-it-yourself surgery, just let me be your nursing back-up."

More Encounters with Surgeons

November 1954, Weston General, Somerset: Hospital #1

I stood rigid in the doorway. She was propped in bed in the surgical ward's only private room. Her faded yellow nightie highlighted her pallor. Her freckled hands rested lightly, so lightly, on the single sheet spread across her tummy. She forced a smile. A single forbidden twelve-year-old tear rolled down my cheek.

The night of her cremation, dreams haunted me. Of the surgeon carving her open like the Christmas turkey, jamming giant fingers into her, grasping those malevolent growths. I heard his voice, resigned, shrugging to his assistant:

"Close her up. Monofilament nylon. I'll check on her tonight."

Did he breathe relief that she was inoperable, saving him hours of toil? Later, did he stand aloof, feign the facts?

Or did he sit at her bedside, clasp her hand? Murmur the truth, the full and awful truth? Wrapping it in words of solace?

He who was as intimate with her entrails as my father with her sex?

*

January 1965, St Bartholomew's, London University: Hospital #2

Fifth year of med school, my initiation to Accident & Emergency. Snow bounced off the fast-flapping plastic doors, the frozen air lifting my skinny half-coat. A&E opened onto Smithfield Meat Market, distribution point of carcasses from Europe's length and breadth for a millennium. It was a twenty-four-seven operation, so the pubs stayed open all night. Outside *The Dog and Duck*, the meat porters had laid down tools. After ten-hour stints of cleaving whole-hogs, tossing half-cows onto massive steel meat hooks, they were downing pints like the fonts were threatening to run dry.

Five AM: an inebriated member of their guild staggered in. His right thumb was dangling where his chopper had sliced it like a twig. He had taken time for a couple more pints of bitter before checking into A&E. What did I recall of the structural attachments of the human pollex? I struggled for fifty minutes to re-oppose the vital organ to its pulped-up palm, knowing my fledgling efforts for a botch. The booze's anesthetic effects endured, though this stoic scion of Agincourt would have conceded no pain were he stone-cold sober.

The staff nurse finally coaxed me to rouse the on-call house surgeon, notorious for his scathing jibes at our woebegone student bunglings, and for his deflowering of nurse probationer virgins. I pressed him on the phone to sally forth grudgingly from his love nest. He dropped one cursory eye upon my handiwork—one misshapen member—and pronounced for all of Smithfield Market to hear:

"Whatever you do, don't take up surgery!"

With this penetrating *bon mot*, and a lustful leer at staff's willowy form in starched white pinafore over Newcastle blue frock, he strutted back to his bower of bliss. Astoundingly, the thumb resumed in time its pristine function, the gaudy jagged wrist-to-index scar a proud memento for both my patient and me.

*

July 1970, Jenny Lind Children's, Norfolk: Hospital #3

My first day of pediatric internship. I took in the higgledy-piggedly scatter of surgical beds. A toddler advanced on me, arms stretched skywards, a study in mute entreaty. How did I get to be twenty-seven and never cradle a child? I dropped to a clumsy kneel, spared a thought for my new three-piece pinstripe. He clambered into my arms and pressed his sticky bib (ice cream? spaghetti loops?) against my old-school tie. The worldly-wise nursing sister ruffled his curls.

"One of your theatre cases for tomorrow, doctor."

Theatre? As in Operating Theatre?

The words—"Whatever you do, don't take up surgery!"—echoed in my ears. She regarded me doubtfully over half-glasses, sensing my concern.

"Circs, my love. Don't look so worried, they'll show you how."

"I thought they did those at birth?"

"Oh, they're much choosier nowadays, dear. Only do the essentials. Phimosis, that sort of thing."

Eight AM: I was the only possible surgeon in sight. Blanking on the requisite scrub time, I soaped from fingertips to armpits for twelve minutes, then pushed backward into the operating room, an initiate at this dance. I sensed some impatience to strike up the band as I took my place at table, contemplated the sleeping tot beneath the gas man's eye.

I felt hands fumbling behind me, twisted my head. Were my trousers slipping down? I breathed relief as the circulating nurse closed my gown, fastened it at waist and neck, and opened the glove wrapper like a book. I grasped and donned the contents. Her scrubbed-in partner was anointing the tiny penis with Betadine and encasing it in sterile green, leaving me a two-inch-square operating field. She handed me a minuscule scalpel, then broke the silence.

"Probably didn't know to expect this. Fear not, I've trained a few interns in my time."

I looked up from contemplating my patient's willy, sensed the smirk beneath the mask, took in the wisp of white hair escaping beneath the cap. Nurses training doctors? Was this even legal?

"You're going to slit his foreskin open, doctor. Right here."

Under her guidance I snipped tentatively along the tiny pecker. "Push back with your fingers, so just his little knob sticks out. The business end, you might say."

Was I cutting off this mite's future pleasure? I sensed a disturbing intimacy between us—this motherly nurse, this little boy's appendage, and me. I complied as she plucked a diminutive plastic ring from her surgical arsenal.

"Now draw the foreskin over this." Her practiced hands continued to guide me. "Now, tie this ligature to staunch the blood when you chop it off. The foreskin, I mean, not the whole organ."

Was she trying to lighten things up? Sweat was trickling down my forehead as I pulled the nylon tight, flashing back to that bloody misshapen thumb. I pictured this little-boy penis and that meat porter-thumb as much of a size. My nurse-mentor handed me pint-sized surgical scissors; I could just squeeze finger and thumb tips through the loops.

"Now, the coup de grace! Lop it off!"

The tiny integument dropped into her waiting basin. She cocooned the remaining member in bandages, just the tip of the meatus peeking out.

"Well done, doctor!"

"Can't claim much credit."

"Nonsense! See one, do one, teach one. You'll be a pro in no time."

*

March 1974, Yorkhill Children's, University of Glasgow: Hospital #4

Come the dawn, I would be delivering my debut lecture to a national jury of my peers—five-hundred members of the British Paediatric Association. Would I sleep tonight? I took up the dog-eared pages of my speech, switched on my portable projector, scanned three years of research: a 276-page doctoral dissertation compressed into twenty slides. I'd got it down word-for-word, but my mind was jerking like washing in a windstorm. I would just run through it once more…

At two-thirty in the morning I dropped into an edgy slumber, replete with dreams of serried ranks in dim lit halls. Over breakfast, a paternal hand dropped onto my acromial process. I twisted my head. Dr. W., our children's surgeon, was grinning at me. A grin like a troll's.

"Ah think I'll gi' tha' wee talk of yoors a miss, Johnnie. I was in the room nex' door, heerd it more than a few times through the early hours. Reckon I could gi' it missen!"

My blush mounted from chest to forehead. Why the hell didn't he bang on the wall and shut me up? Did he lose his beauty sleep simply to make a monkey of me over my eggs and bacon? With a light clap on my scapula, he was gone, leaving me to sally forth, stand before the podium and strive to wow the hallowed hordes.

*

January 1979, Rainbow Babies & Children's, Case Western Reserve University: Hospital #5

"High-grad osteo. Biopsy confirms it."

My first encounter with Dr. M., our orthopedist: he tapped his forefinger on the telltale lesion on the Xray screen. I read her name off the film: Brandy. The cancer had totally replaced this fourteen-year-old's humeral head and extended halfway down the shaft.

"But this girlie has an unusual problem. Been deaf from birth, relies entirely on sign language. Amputation's the gold standard, of course. But what's your experience with limb salvage? You've got good drugs to shrink these bastards, don't you?"

Limb salvage: a new way to avoid amputation for bone cancers in the young. I'd only read about it. It had become dubbed neoadjuvant chemotherapy: to start the chemo right at the outset to shrink the cancer enough for the surgeon to resect the remainder without having to remove the limb.

"I've never done one. But yes, we could give the chemo upfront, make your job easier, maybe even save her hand. You leaning that way?"

"All for it, if you're game."

I felt a flush of excitement. "I'd love to try it. Have you talked to her family?"

"Briefly. If your drugs work, I'll resect the thing *in toto*, insert a titanium implant, reattach her arm to her shoulder. Bingo."

I was warming to him, wondering what made him tick. Could we chat over coffee? Do surgeons chat—or just make a virtue of eternal busyness? He was heading for the door. Over his shoulder, "They're checking into clinic in the morning. See you there."

*

Dr. M. stood silent in the window as I examined Brandy. Her arm's tumescence stretched from shoulder to elbow, mirroring the X-rays. I eyed the sheen of dread coating her face, hazarded a smile, then turned to Mom.

"Mrs. Andrews, you understand Brandy's condition? And the possible treatments?"

"Yes, doctor. Usually you'd…take away her arm. Amputate." She stumbled over the word, her eyes damp, her words hanging dense in the air. "But you could give Brandy your drugs first, then you mightn't have to?"

"Yes, that's what we're hoping. But we've never had anyone in Brandy's… situation. And it's a very new form of treatment, we can't make promises. It may not work well enough to save her hand. How does Brandy communicate—with both hands?"

Mom swallowed, fixed her look upon her daughter. Had Brandy been lip-reading all this?

"Perhaps she could learn to use just her left. But it would be like a whole new language." She brought the backs of two knuckles to her eyes to wipe away tears. "Do you want me to ask her?"

"Yes, I'd very much like to know what Brandy thinks."

The signing went back and forth between them for long minutes, neither hiding their distress. Mom turned back to me.

"It'd be hard, doctor, very hard." She glanced at Dr. M. as though to draw him in. He nodded silent affirmation. "But we want you to try."

"Thank you, Mrs. Andrews. I'm sorry to upset you both. This is a very hard time." I leaned back in my chair. "We'll get the chemo started right off. You can stay with Brandy."

*

Two months and four chemo courses later, Brandy's shoulder and upper arm had shrunk to almost normal size. She could use both hands to brush her hair—what little was left of it. I'd learned a few sign words and letters, though I couldn't translate the sounds she made. Two weeks after the last course, Dr. M. called me again. I headed downstairs at the double to where he was once more peering at the screen.

"Better than I'd hoped. The whole deal looks dead as potato chips. I'm putting her on my list for Thursday."

I gaped at the films, dumbstruck. "Next Thursday. Yes, sure. Her counts are back up, and everything else is good."

Four days later, Brandy's arm was encased in a cast from shoulder to wrist, her fingers swollen to twice their normal size. But she was signing to Mom with both hands. And I had read the path report: One hundred-percent necrotic bone.

*

December 1985, Shands, University of Florida: Hospital # 6

Dr. D dialed back the lumens on the 'scope. I could no longer hold my eye open. He could no longer see anything through my tears.

“I don’t know what the heck I’m looking at, John. Infection, for sure, but it beats me what. You wear contacts?”

“Yeah, till last week. Not anymore—can’t go near them.” My eyes were clamped shut against the glaring overhead lamp.

“Sorry, I’ll dim it. Photophobia’s hell.” We sat together in shadow. He laid a hand on my arm. “Your contacts could be the culprit. I’ll see you back daily till I nail it. Real sorry you’re hurting, man. We’ve got good eye patches, better than Walmart’s. And anesthetic drops, along with the antibiotics. I’ll get you all you need.”

Thanks, doctor. For laying on your hand. For saying, *I don’t know.*

*

Acanthamoeba keratitis. The diagnosis took him two weeks. Fourteen days of studying photos in every tome he could lay his hands on. Of consulting colleagues across the country. Of having every member of the Ophthalmology faculty check me out. He tried one eye drop after another, finally settled for PHMB[1] and Brolene. He told me I was the first to get this combination. Then the eye bank in Atlanta called.

“They’ve got a cornea for you, John. It’ll be here tomorrow. I’m admitting you *stat*, stepping up the drops to hourly.”

I woke through twilight anaesthesia, reached my arms up through the haze to hug him. Grinned idiotically at my goof. “Thought you were Sheila,” my voice slurred.

“I talked to her.” His face was close, inspecting his handiwork. “No sign of the parasite, man.”

I was back at work two weeks later. I’d been certain I would lose my eye, that the infection would spread to the other side, that I’d be blind, that I’d never work again.

Thanks, Bill.

*

May 1995, Yale-New Haven: Hospital # 7

Lunching with Dr. S. at his wife's off-campus café.

"I've got time to sit and chat, now I'm retired. When I'm not bussing and loading dishes." His voice was a light caress. "I had to do it. At fifty-eight, I was getting up at four a.m. to pen a few pages before heading to work. So—no more operating for me, just writing about them. And other things."

Later at my lecture I read them the poem about speaking truth to children. How I'd told Joey, an eight-year-old with dreadfully widespread cancer, that he was going to die. How his parents had wanted him to know, wanted no conspiracy of silence between the three of them. How his Mom had approached me, diffident but resolute: "Could you tell Joey, doctor?" How Joey had howled for three long minutes at the finality of my words. How he had spied Mom's tears, and mine, stopped his own on an in-breath. How he'd gone on to play the stand-up comic, offer his wry observation on my messy office: "Didn't your mom teach you to pick up after yourself?"

Did my candour free him to run this gamut of emotion? And was that good? Afterwards, you approached me. "Sorry—I couldn't do that. Surgeons are really softies, you know. Tell the truth but tell it slant, that's me. My failure perhaps."

Confessions of a knife?[2]

He added, his soft tones beguiling, free of accusation, "Perhaps you worked up to it?"

"Yes. Yes, I beat about the bush a bit. Before I came to it."

Thank you, Richard. No softie, you. Just a gentle man.

Dear Surgeons,

You arouse in me awe, diffidence, unease. Thirty years a professor, in your presence I am once more the callow twelve-year-old. Your tight-lipped competence daunts me. You relish thinking on your feet; something I stumble over. I am a klutz with a scalpel; you can stand ten hours for a Whipple[3], feet no longer your own, taking silent pride in those endless hours.

[1]*Polyhexamethylene Biguanide (Baquacil).*

[2]Richard Seltzer (1979). *Confessions of a Knife.* Simon & Schuster.

[3]*Pancreaticoduodenectomy*—the Whipple procedure.

To Operate or Not To...

"He's on a ventilator in the PICU, John. I don't think he's got long."

I had just bumped into our pediatric neurosurgeon in the hospital atrium coffee line. I mentioned that I'd recently started up a pediatric palliative care service and he told me about this patient I might like to see.

"The whole family came from Puerto Rico, pretty much looking for miracles. Their two-year-old has Larsen's Syndrome. It's a pretty rare inherited disorder which causes all kinds of problems. His dorsal and cervical spine are so badly buckled it's almost impossible for the little guy to breathe on his own. And he's got several dislocated joints—elbows, hips, knees, bilateral club feet. All kinds of trouble. His mom just had to make a real hard decision about my not operating on his spine. I think maybe she was right."

The unit clerk directed me and Marilyn, my nurse, to Mateo's room. His mom, Camila, was kneeling beside the crib, cooing to him through the bars. It seemed doubtful the boy knew she was there, given that he was full of opioids and Ativan for his unremitting pain. But who was I to judge? They say sometimes fully anaesthetized people can be aware of their surroundings. And no doubt Camila had been offering Mateo similar soothing sounds ever since he was still in her womb.

Much of the little boy's face and upper body were hidden behind the paraphernalia of intensive care, but we could still make out his badly buckled spine and short bent legs. He must have been born into pain, and never been free of it. I introduced myself to Camila and explained why I was here. That I was especially experienced with relieving pain and anxiety in both children and their families, and that I could be a listening ear for someone far from home.

"Maybe you'd like to talk about things."

"Thank you, Doctor."

Camila rose to her feet, a handsome Hispanic woman in her late twenties with a straight-on look. Her husband, Angelo, moved quietly behind her as I guided them into the social worker's room. Once settled in a comfy chair, Camila held us rapt with her son's story, speaking in almost fluent English with only a trace of Hispanic accent.

"When I first took him home from the hospital, I shut us both up in our spare room for five days, so I could learn how to feed him around his cleft palate, scoop up his higgledy-piggledy arms and legs, and cuddle him like they showed me in the hospital. I fell in love with him, Doctor." Her face took on an almost defiant look. "The priest at St Domingo's, he told me the problems Mateo was born with were punishment for my sins. I'll never go back to that church again.

"So I packed us all up—Mateo and my husband and Tomas, my three-year-old—and we took the plane to New York. I had heard that was where we would find the best surgeon to help my son. It has been especially hard on my husband—he has his engineering business in San Juan, but he has had to let that go. All he can find here is part time work on a building site for minimum wage. Well, if it rains, he gets to stay home with us."

She offered this almost as an afterthought, while Angelo sat quietly on the window seat as she told her story.

"This specialist, he spent maybe five minutes examining Mateo, then he moved away and talked to his nurse, never to me. I think she was Puerto Rican, too. The guy waited while she translated everything into Spanish—I never got a chance to tell him I understood exactly what he was saying. It all happened too quickly. He simply told his nurse, 'No way I'm going to touch this case,' which she translated to me as, 'The doctor's sorry, but he doesn't feel he can operate on your baby.' But he never mentioned anything, not even to the nurse, about why he wouldn't even try."

Camila's eyes were glistening as she struggled to hold back tears. Marilyn handed her the box of tissues from the table.

"So afterwards, when the surgeon had gone, his nurse talked to me some more. She told me not to give up hope. She had heard from a friend in Miami that there was a very good brain surgeon here at the University of Florida. She gave me his name, so I moved us all down here. Well, he may not have a big name like that other doctor, but he listened to me, and he talked to me. He said things like he could see what a good mom I was and how supportive my husband was. And he gave me a chance to *choose*."

Camila stopped talking again, as though gathering her energy to keep going. "But he told me about the big risks if he operated. He said Mateo could very well be paralyzed after the surgery on his spine. And he would have to drill holes in his skull to fasten some kind of metal halo, he called it, to keep his neck from dislocating. He said Mateo would need twelve months of traction, maybe, and that he would be in pain most of that time. How he could easily get infections, even in his brain.

"It all sounded just too frightening, but at least he told us everything that could happen. Well, right now Mateo can wave his arms and smile, and he seems pretty happy as long as he has medicine for his pain. My husband and I, we talked, and we decided: Mateo should have as happy a life as he can, even if it is just for a short time. We don't want him to go through months of suffering, maybe for no good in the end."

Camila seemed at peace with her choice. Her husband was nodding his agreement. He clearly understood most of what his wife had said, although she was obviously the decision-maker in the family. At least in matters of life and death—as they were now having to face together.

"No matter what, he's in God's hands," were her last words to us as we left her beside Mateo's crib.

But the next day when Marilyn and I got back to the PICU, we were astonished to find Mateo was no longer on a ventilator. Unknown to us, Dr. S. had gone ahead and ordered one more MRI—"Just to see how much more his cord is compressed," he said later. We caught up with Camila at Mateo's bedside. He was still fast asleep, but he was now free of most of his intensive care impedimenta, apart from a tight-fitting oxygen mask and the standard monitoring equipment.

"I have changed my mind," she told us, once Marilyn and I had pulled up our chairs. "The surgeon said the MRI hadn't got any worse over the last couple of months, so he thinks Mateo has a real chance after all." She paused. "He went over all the risks again, but he felt it was definitely worth an attempt.

"Then I knew it was really up to me—my husband would go along with whatever I decided. If I said no, Mateo would most likely die while he was still in here." She glanced around at the sterile atmosphere of the ICU. "And if I told him to go ahead with the surgery, I would be committing him—all of us—to maybe a year camped out in this hospital. And that would be just to get his neck fixed. After that he would need a whole lot more surgeries on his arms and legs. Recently he has been so happy. Playing and smiling, moving his legs and arms—he won't be able to do any of these things for months and months, maybe never, if he has *the surgery*."

She repeated the last two words and rolled her eyes up and to the right each time she said them. It was clear that she was still feeling her guilt. The operation would cause Mateo great and lasting pain, and he could still be dead very soon anyway. How would she live with that? She was scared, too, about how she would manage to take care of him, if he was largely paralyzed but lingered on.

But she had seen it clearly: this was her son's one chance for a full life. He must already be feeling the weight of his disability: condemned to lie face-up in his bed for long hours, watching his brother playing. She couldn't bear the idea of sending Tomas back to his grandparents in Puerto Rico during Mateo's long recovery; she had already watched their lives grow farther and farther apart. She wondered, too, how her husband would cope. The work opportunities were so few, and he was much more alienated by American culture.

What would any of us have decided? It's hard to think of a greater sacrifice for Mateo's whole family than the many surgeries he could be facing. What is it about mortal life that we are willing to take such chances, accept such pain? Is it so precious? And where could this Catholic family find faith, and a God to pray to, after what the Puerto Rican priest had told her.

But by next morning, Camila had talked to her husband, had prayed silently to this God she was no longer sure of. And she had made her decision: they would go ahead with the surgery. It would be many months, after the last of Mateo's several surgeries to straighten his spine and decompress his cord, the huge metal halo still Jerry-rigged to his back brace, before he was able to sit up and look around him for the first time. He would still need the orthopedic surgeons to go to work on his dislocated elbows, hips, knees, and his severely clubbed feet.

But for now, he could swallow tasty morsels of food, and he could play with his brother. The choice had been made; Mateo had a real chance of becoming a schoolboy, even of growing to adulthood. The last time we saw him—six months after our very first visit—the little boy was in a much simpler brace and was able to sit up enough to look about him freely, to eat meals, and to play freely with his toys and with his brother Tomas.

Risks

Sometimes you get thanked for something you can claim no real credit for. One cold and dreary February day, I finished up early morning attending rounds with the pediatric residents and medical students and made my solitary way up to the pediatric intensive care unit on the tenth floor. As I came through the double doors, Ryan's mother hurled herself upon me.

Maybe she had memorized my daily schedule and knew exactly when to expect me. She was as tall as I was, and heavier by a good bit. I all but lost my balance and toppled backwards onto the floor, with her on top. It was only some kind of Aikido move as I gave way before her that saved us both. Regaining my footing, and my senses, I felt as much as heard the sobs rising up out of her chest. I spread my legs to get a better purchase and we hung onto each other. We held this position for at least a minute, both of us breathless from the sudden encounter. She was trying to get on top of her long aching sobs, while I was wondering what was coming next, and what I was going to do about it.

Over the past six months, I had come to know this woman, along with her toddler son, about as well as any of us had. Even the nurses didn't use her first name, as is the custom with the mothers of most of our cancer patients. Up until now she had stayed impassive, almost taciturn, in the face of all the setbacks that had overtaken Ryan, along with my inadequate attempts to explain them. She had certainly never let loose with tears before, so I had a pretty good idea how long she had been hanging on to them.

The first time we had met was just after Ryan's first birthday. She had taken him to his pediatrician when she noticed that he'd had almost no wet diapers for the past three days. She had watched him trying to pee when she was bathing him; he could manage only a dribble, far from the once robust stream that would often catch her on the receiving end. Then she realized his lower belly was swollen well beyond its normal tubbiness. By the time she had made it to the doctor's office, she had to have been seriously frightened. But it was not in her nature to show it.

The pediatrician had felt a hard mass across his abdomen that seemed to be rising up from deep in his pelvis. Within a day of his sending Ryan on to the university medical center, we had the answer. Blood tests that afternoon told us his kidneys were failing fast, and a CAT scan of his belly gave us the rest of the story. There was a craggy lump growing forward from the back of his lower spine; it was this that was obstructing the flow of urine out of his bladder. The build-up of urine was in turn putting back pressure on his ureters, and his kidneys were swollen to more than twice their proper size, a condition we call hydronephrosis. Those kidneys were dying fast.

We could comfort ourselves that at least the cancer hadn't invaded his spinal cord to cause paralysis below it. Ryan could kick his legs back and forth as vigorously as any normal one-year-old. We had aborted the immediate threat to Ryan's life by hooking him up to a dialysis machine, to take over the work of the kidneys and clear the build-up of waste from his bloodstream. His mother didn't visit much during this time; she had two other children under seven at home, and her youngest was spending his time too heavily sedated to show much distress at her absence.

Between two episodes of dialysis, each of which was an almost day-long procedure, one of our pediatric surgeons took Ryan to the operating room for a biopsy of the cancer that was spreading across the bottom of his little belly. It turned out to be a rarity, even allowing for the scarcity of any kind of malignant growth in children. This one—Ewing's sarcoma—usually invades the bones of the arms and legs and pelvis of teenagers. Even then, Ewing's sarcoma accounts for about one percent of children's cancers, so both Ryan's age and the location of his cancer made him distinctly unusual. As with almost every childhood cancer, no one has found out why on earth this happens. One of my senior partners told me, "It's just another act of God that it hasn't been given to us to figure out."

Maybe he was right. But if the origin of such an awful event remains a mystery, there is some balance in the universe. Our very earthly pharmacy has been blessed with an array of chemotherapy that the robust healing systems of young children can handle a whole lot better than the average adult. Some have been synthesized by chemists and pharmacologists from their grassroots elements; many more have come to light by chance, and by divine inspiration. Perhaps God really does work through doctors.

One look at his CAT scan told the surgeon it would be impossible for her to peel this cancerous mass off the front of Ryan's lumbosacral spine without doing untold damage to the vital complex of nerves that arises out of the spinal cord. But we found out some years back that many childhood cancers respond so well to our chemo that surgeons usually allow us to have the first shot. Neoadjuvant therapy, as it's termed, can usually shrink a cancerous mass down to a much more operable size and make the job of resecting it a whole lot easier. When we had finished our initial X-rays and blood tests and found no sign of the cancer spreading to distant parts of Ryan's body, we breathed a collective sigh of relief and set about our chemotherapy.

As with almost every young child, Ryan bounced back to life after two rounds of chemo over the next couple of weeks. Unlike his mother, he was a sparky little one who quickly got to enjoy the attention. Suddenly he had a bunch of moms in the persons of our nurses—and one or two extra dads—whom he quickly won over. Meanwhile, his mother would appear at odd times, sit with him for an hour or so, never seek us out with queries or comments, then slip away as quietly as she had arrived.

Within weeks, the cancer started to shrink, and the pressure on his bladder and kidneys eased. After two months, and several rounds of the drugs, the mass was a quarter of its original size on the CAT scan, and Ryan was toddling to greet me when he came to my clinic for check-ups. The problem, though, was that his kidneys were still not behaving themselves. His bladder and ureters had a pretty twisted look to them and were still not letting his urine flow free. As a result, the function of his kidneys was far from normal. After some debate our surgeon decided further surgery was needed—this time to try to correct his internal anatomy. His mother took this news, like everything else, with stoicism.

"Do what's best," was all she said.

"What about his dad?" I asked her. "Don't you want to talk it over with him?"

"He's gone. Good riddance."

This was the first I had heard of a break-up. It must have happened since their son got sick. I realized that the only time I had met Ryan's dad was for a few brief minutes when we first broke the news of his son's illness.

"Well, he'll want to know what's going on, won't he? I think he ought to know."

"I don't know where he's at. Off in the woods with his gun most likely."

Disappearing dads are a not uncommon outcome of cancer in the young. This was by no means the first time I had run into parents who couldn't hold it together under the strain of an illness that threatened the life of their child. Ryan's mother remained impassive behind the barrier she had erected between us. Whenever I tried to get a little closer and draw her out, she would retreat into her physical and emotional shell. This was her way of dealing with the world and all its mischief. Frustrating as it was to us caregivers, it was not our job to try to change this lifelong pattern.

Once the surgeon opened up his abdominal cavity once more, she found everything inside Ryan's pelvis to be scarred and matted down. It was clear she wasn't going to be able to dig the remaining cancerous tissue out without putting all those vital nerves and blood vessels at great risk. She did manage to unravel most of the little boy's pelvic tissues, realigning them and making sure the connections between his kidneys, ureters, and bladder were free and clear.

“Hope those suckers stay open this time,” she muttered over a quick cup of coffee when she recounted to me what she had found.

Ryan bounced back once more from the effects of this second surgery—the miraculous way very young ones do. He was up and about again in four days, home in a week. Then we weighed in once more with our chemo drugs, this time adding a modest dose of radiation treatment to try to kill off the remaining cancer cells without damaging anything else beyond repair. I no longer quizzed his mother about how she was doing, how things were at home. We would exchange a word, a look, a nod—but nothing more.

The nurses met the same taciturn reception, but no one questioned her dedication to her young family. She might not be saying much, but she kept up her pattern of turning up bang on time in the clinic for her son’s treatment, often with her other two children in tow. These two were always clean and well-dressed, but as unforthcoming as their mother. I thought about their dad out there in the woods, nursing his gun and no doubt his guilt. These young ones had learned silence well.

The cancer stayed shrunken down to a fraction of its original size, but Ryan’s X-rays and blood tests kept telling us his kidneys were still not back to their normal working order. We worried that our treatment, especially the radiation doses, would start to do more harm than good. The long-term effects of our cancer therapies are not as dramatic as the immediate ones, but they are more worrisome because of their possible permanence. We have learned over the years how we could cure many of our children of their cancers, only to have their kidneys, or liver, or even their heart, give out some years down the line. Not the greatest trade-off.

We walked this tightrope for three more months. A further set of X-rays told us the cancer was all but gone, but at the expense of Ryan’s normal pelvic anatomy and the health of his kidneys. Leaving the hospital that evening by the entrance most of the patients and their families use, I spotted his mother puffing on a Marlboro Light in one of the smoking areas ringing the hospital. She always sat off to the side, seeming to take no pleasure in the company of her fellow smokers. I approached her tentatively; by now I felt like a stalker.

"He's going to need more surgery to straighten things out down there."

She said nothing.

"It's touch and go. We've done as much as we can. It's in the hands of the surgeon to see if she can set things to rights. His kidneys are still a lot bigger than they should be."

"Do what you gotta."

"It might not make any difference. His kidneys may never work quite right. He's still a little tyke and he's only got a little space down there. There's a lot of scarring, too. We think it's a chance we should take, though …"

I trailed off, wishing I could get some reaction out of her.

"Better get on with it then."

The next morning Ryan went back into surgery for the third time. If anything, the appearances were worse: more scars tethering down bladder, ureters, nerves, blood vessels. A harder and harder field for the surgeon to work in. This time our pediatric surgeon had called in a urologist to help, a surgeon specializing in the particular problems of the urinary and genital systems. Together, they painstakingly dissected the layers of tissue bound down to the front of Ryan's sacrum at the very base of his spine, trying once more to create free and safe passage for his urine flow and relieve the back pressure that was slowly wearing his kidneys out. They had done all they could; it was in God's hands.

Three days later I got the news. I was on my way to see Ryan in the PICU where he was recuperating, having checked on his latest blood report and X-ray findings. For the first time since I had met this little boy, his blood work showed his kidneys were in perfect working order. And the new X-rays suggested that they were already getting smaller, a sign that the back pressure was at last easing off. I gave thanks to God, and to the enormous skills of my surgical colleagues.

It was then that I encountered his mother as I came through the PICU doors. I was quite unprepared for her reaction, for the final bursting of her dam of tears. After holding on tight for many months to every emotional bone in her body, it took the best news yet to finally open the floodgates. The exchange of energies between two people—physical, emotional, spiritual—is powerful healing medicine.

Standing there in my Aikido stance, I took a deep breath. Before I could help it, I found myself inhaling the strong savour of Marlboro Lites. I tried not to flinch as I looked beyond her at Ronnie, Ryan's nurse, standing behind her. We raised mute eyebrows. I caught sight of her little one through the glass door of the isolation unit, slumbering peaceably under his Pooh Bear blanket. Between shallower breaths, and with my head averted, I entertained irreverent thoughts about passive smoke and the hazards of health care.

Ryan's mom was still gripping me tight; I could feel her snuffles moistening the shoulder of my white coat. I groped about in my right-hand pocket for my supply of grubby tissues and wedged them between us. She loosened her grip enough to reach for them, wipe and blow her nose, and stare red-eyed at me. Then her face crumpled again, and I started to guide her backwards in a slow dance through the swinging ICU doors. It felt like she was my first date, and this was the last dance of the evening.

We weaved towards the two rocking chairs reposing together in the passage behind the doors. Now I was envisioning myself easing my date off the dance floor and outdoors onto the patio. The chairs had an unused look, the wood of their broad arms still gleaming. They had been a present to the unit last Christmas, I remembered, from Beth Rose's family. Beth Rose had spent months on a ventilator after a near-drowning accident that no one thought she would come through, but she had finally graduated to the hospital's step-down unit. As Ryan's mother drew away from me, the smell of passive smoke grew stronger. I thought about her two other children; they must have been breathing in these stale fumes all their lives. The harmful effects would already be there to see in their bronchial linings.

Then I caught myself: what right had I to make such judgments? Did I have three under-sevens, one with cancer, to raise single-handed? She loosened her grip on me a little more, and we sank onto the polished wood. My back and shoulders were aching from holding both her and myself upright. I rested my weight against the chair's support, and my attention wandered. I could hear the voices about us—of chattering humanity moving up and down the corridor, in and out of the unit. Orderlies maneuvering gurneys on which young ones lay sleeping, medical students and pediatric residents scurrying to rounds or to answer pages, nurses idling back from lunch breaks, families returning for visiting hour. It didn't matter; she wasn't hearing any of it.

I slid my arm around the back of her chair and rocked it gently. I thought for a moment that she had fallen asleep, she was so still. Then she leant toward me again, pushed her forehead against my upper ribs.

"Thanks, Doc."

"Hey, it's those surgeons you've got to thank. They did all the work."

"Yeah. Thanks, anyway."

Maybe I was just in the right place at the right time. But somehow I couldn't see this mother clutching my surgical colleagues in her arms. We doctors aren't always too good at accepting compliments; I decided this was the time for graceful acceptance.

Part Six

Living and Dying

First Physical

St Paul's Cathedral clock was striking nine on July 1, 1963, as I entered the hallowed sanctum of Barts Hospital. In 1123—more than eight-hundred years earlier—Rahere the Monk, courtier to Henry II, had swung open the hospital's West Gates onto Giltspur Street in the City of London to usher in London's plague-ridden hordes. None of those original twelve-inch-thick walls still stood, but the primeval austerity of the place endured. A raw twenty-two-year-old medical student, I was shaking in my shiny lace-up shoes.

I peeked my head around the door of Annie Zunz ward, knowing better than to enter without Sister's permission. Sister Annie Zunz was sitting bolt upright at her desk facing directly away from me, starched apron stretched over dark blue ankle-length dress. To left and right of her sat a staff nurse like two ministering angels at the side of God. I cleared my throat and asked permission to enter the ward. The conversation broke off; the white veil-cap inclined forward brief inches. I took this for assent. The ward stretched ahead of me, two lines of beds as spick and span and precisely spaced as an army barracks awaiting the brigadier's inspection. The patients mostly lay recumbent and immobile, as though loath to disturb the apple-pie order. I counted mutely as I ventured forward, clutching the admission chart of my new assignment. I knew her earlier medical charts would take several days to appear from some dusty hospital records repository. All I had was her name, address (somewhere in London's docklands) and D.O.A. (date of admission) to work with.

Oh God, was it seven or seventeen? I was almost at the far end of the ward before I located my patient by surreptitiously reading off the name at the end of each bed. (A strict no-no to seek out the names of people other than my own patient). I recalled my house officer's recent admonition that I would need a chaperone before carrying out my P.E.—physical examination—but it seemed safe enough to get rolling with the H.P.C.—history of present condition—until Sister Annie Zunz saw fit to free up a probationer nurse for the lowly task of guarding her charges against possible medical student improprieties.

I sensed Mrs. Lovell had been awaiting my arrival. She proved ancient and frail and was propped up on no fewer than four pillows. Could this be an early clue—did she have trouble breathing if she laid down flat? Remembering the house officer's injunction not to stand and loom over my patient, I eased her fresh bed linen from the chair onto the crowded bedside table to make room for me to sit. I laid my H.&P.—history and physical—aide-memoir on my lap and remembered to introduce myself by proffering my hand. As she extended her own, I caught myself naming the linear humps of her forearm bones so readily visible beneath the papery skin. They danced some kind of *port de bras* as her wrist rotated and her fingers grasped mine: live anatomy displayed before me as though springing from the dog-eared pages of my recently discarded *Cunningham's Manual of Practical Anatomy.*

Which is the radius and which the ulna? Is that pronation or supination? Are those metacarpals or phalanges? But I had left my hard-won anatomy gleanings alongside that manual in Professor Cave's dissection rooms. What possible relevance could they have to my present ponderings? As my hand enveloped Mrs. Lovell's—a meshwork of tiny, quite unnamable bones—a tremor passed between us. Was it hers or mine? The house officer's mandate to hold eye contact was ringing in my ears, precluding my peeking at the list of questions on my clipboard. I scrawled notes blindly as my patient unravelled her story. I was swiftly cast adrift from the prescribed order of my H.&P, powerless to staunch the flow as she recounted each minute detail of her family circumstances.

"Not that I mind bein' 'ere, Doc, but it's me pussycat. Me ol' man makes sure to give 'er 'er kibble, like, but 'e don't 'old wiv changin' 'er litter box. It's allus a 'orrid mess when I gets 'ome. Oh, you're not a doctor yet, though, are you, I can always tell, well, student doctor then, same difference is what I allus say."

As her chatter gained momentum, I deferred all attempts to sort my clipboard scribblings until I could find a quiet spot—though where that might be amidst these alien surroundings totally eluded me. I registered the arrival of the promised probationer nurse, who was engaged in pulling the ceiling-to-floor curtains around to conceal the three of us from the outside world. I was still well short on the many components of my R.O.S.—Review of Systems—having completed only three: cardiovascular, respiratory, and E.N.T. Questions regarding Mrs. Lovell's gastrointestinal, neurological, and musculoskeletal health still lay ahead, and when and how to fit in her P.M.H., F.H. and S.H.—past medical history, family history, and social history—I would have to leave to providence.

This would be my one and only chance to avail myself of this nurse's services before she was whisked away on far more pressing duties. One glance told me she had to be straight out of high school and wouldn't say boo to a goose. But it was high time to move full speed ahead to the clinical exam. Did either of my companions have any notion that Mrs. L. was my first live patient? I stood up to carry out my P.E., knowing I had to conduct it from the right side of the patient's bed. I wondered briefly if any exceptions were made for left-handers? And why must one sit for history-takings but stand for physical examinations?

I was forced to pause every few minutes to visualize the items on my P.E. list, but it was quickly clear that my patient was far more familiar with the routine than me. She anticipated my every request and responded without demur. I pulled my brand new flashlight from my pristine white coat pocket and gazed into Mrs. L.'s mouth. After several long-drawn-out moments of flashing and peering, I learned only that she had but one tooth remaining from the set with which God had once blessed her. I limited my eye exam to checking for reactions and rotations, having forgotten to tote along my brand new ophthalmoscope. Its absence was no big loss, given that I hardly knew how to switch it on, let alone tap into its diagnostic powers.

I fumbled to capture the thready pulse at her wrist, remembering to turn her head gently away from me so that I could study the carotid artery in its steady up-

and-down rhythm motion above her thoracic inlet. As I observed this conspicuous motion, I realized I had no clue about the appearance of this impulse: was it normal or not? And if not, what on earth did it signify? As I was locating the second hand on my watch to count her wrist pulse, the beating artery slipped swiftly from beneath my fingers. Despite Mrs. L.'s gratifying compliance, my H.&P. had so far failed to offer a single tip-off as to what might have brought her in here.

I glanced at the nurse, standing mute and patient at the other side of the bed—and took in for the first time how utterly ravishing she was. Her thick copper-coloured hair was pulled back tightly under her cap above the face of an angel. Her devastating prettiness, in such contrast to the ancient Mrs. Lovell, was stirring me to the core. I tried furtively to read off the name on her badge, bringing me in direct line of sight of her right breast. Blushing, I averted my eyes as she turned her attention to folding the sheets down. I swiveled my mind back to the job in hand as she helped Mrs. L. with the straps of her yellow flannel nightgown. It promptly dropped to her waist, and I took in the thin arc of ribs jutting out from the sides of her breastbone. The years had left their mark on every inch of Mrs. L., her skin a discoloured mass of blotches and wrinkles, paper-thin to my touch. Her breasts were dappled with brown marks like fallen leaves, blue venules crisscrossing their almost flat translucent surface.

How old was she, anyway? Eighty? Ninety? How could I have I missed such a glaring detail? I became aware of the growing ache in my braced legs but felt too shy to perch on the edge of my half-naked patient's bed. I remembered just in time to rub the end of my virgin stethoscope up and down on my pristine white coat to take the chill off the metal. As the nurse delicately lifted up Mrs. L's left breast, I spotted the brief upward movement of what had to be her cardiac apex. I laid first bell, then diaphragm, over it, tuning into gushes and murmurs that till this moment had been only stark words in *Cecil & Loeb's Textbook of Medicine*.

I glanced surreptitiously at my cheat sheet. My mind was a blank. A single row of words leapt out: *inspection, palpation, percussion, auscultation*—look, feel, sound, listen. Hell, I had totally skipped percussion—that business about flattening my left hand against her chest and tapping right middle and ring fingers against left middle, to try to determine if there was anything else in her lungs besides air. Anything that shouldn't be there, that is. I offered up silent thanks that both patient and nurse were ready for my next move. The probationer was supporting Mrs. L. as she leant forward in the bed. I laid my palm flat over her left shoulder blade, trying to keep my overlong fingernails from penetrating the fragile skin. I started my tap-tap-tapping on the left middle finger with my right middle and ring ones and was rewarded with a hollow resonance indicating a nice clear lung cavity. I moved my hand downwards and repeated the performance, with the same satisfying result: resonance all the way to the bottom of her lung.

I switched to the right side. All was well until tap-tap-tap number three. It yielded a thud as dull as a stone. Hallelujah, surely something was amiss. I murmured my mantra once more—inspect, palpate, percuss, auscultate …

"Breathe deep and slow, Mrs. Lovell, I'm just going to listen in."

I worked my stethoscope down her back. Sure enough, midway down on the right side, all sounds of in-and-out air movement abruptly vanished. I pulled my stethoscope from my ears; Mrs. L. had once more broken her silence.

"It ain't me lungs, doctor, nuffin' wrong with 'em. It's me liver. It's swellin' up and dahn and all abaht. Cop a feel for yusself."

A piece of information beyond the price of rubies.

The nurse removed all but one pillow and eased Mrs. L. down to a supine posture, then folded her nightie and sheets down to her groin. The fullness and roundness of my patient's tummy leapt out at me, in striking contrast to the scrawniness of the rest of her. My mind struggled to recall the primary causes of an overly protuberant abdomen. She for sure didn't qualify for obesity. And I could safely rule out pregnancy—couldn't I? So all I needed now was to work my way through *Cecil & Loeb's* other twenty-plus causes.

But Mrs. L. had already started to clue me in. I laid a tentative hand over where her liver should be, started to slide it downwards, and had almost reached her groin before my pinkie abutted against something. A firm, thick lip that had to be her liver's bottom edge.

"Feel it, dearie, do you? Big bugger, in'it?"

"Yes, er, yes, it is … er, big."

As I continued my groping, I took in what had to be puncture marks, clustered in a line just below and to the left of her liver edge. Having broken her silence, Mrs. L. was becoming a veritable treasure trove of priceless prompts.

"I spec' they'll be 'aving you stick a needle or two in me, if you're goin' to be me new doctor. "

It took me a long moment to absorb the significance of her words.

"You mean you've had other students putting needles in your tummy, then, Mrs. Lovell?"

"Oh, dearie, yus, plen'y."

"Er, you wouldn't have any idea why, would you? By any possible chance?"

"Why, bless me, yus! Thought you'd never ask, love. Like I said, it's me liver, it may be a big 'un, but it ain't workin' worth tuppence nowadays. Ever since the 'epatitis. So I get all this water in me belly—'scuse me, dear, I mean me tummy."

The penny finally clanged to the floor. I peered more closely at the colour of her skin. Yellow as custard! How could I have missed it? Not what you'd call golden, but—no doubt about it—she was lemon all over. Had to be her nightie that had masked it. Struggling to curb my glee, I turned my scrutiny back to her eyes, lowering each eyelid for a better look. The white parts weren't white at all but lemony too. I was growing giddy at the thought of how close I'd come to missing the glaring signs that Mrs. L's liver was failing fast. Maybe she had a few more vital clues to uncover? Why in God's name didn't I think to ask her what was wrong in the first place? Mrs. L. seemed to have read my thoughts.

"You'll be tellin' the perfessor all about me case in the mornin', then? 'E'll be sure to want to 'ear about me bleedin'."

"Bleeding?"

"Oh yus, that's wot brought me in 'ere this time. I was bringin' up all this blood, and I got to feelin' real giddy, I did. Me old man 'ad to ring up for an ambulance. They said if 'e'd 'ave left it any longer, I might not be 'ere at all. They 'ad to empty me stummich out an' gimme a blood transfusion. They think it's stopped nah. The bleedin', that is."

I glanced back up at the nurse. I had almost forgotten her in my elation.

"Er, nurse, I don't think I'll need you to chaperone me anymore. I'm just going to chat with Mrs. Lovell, see what else she thinks I ought to know."

Did I catch her smirking? Well, perhaps we'll get to chat some more about Mrs. Lovell's case. Now wouldn't that be nice …

"'Ere, I wouldn't mind sittin' back up again," Mrs. L. interrupted my reverie. "Gets me quite aht of breath, lyin' down does."

The two of us moved fast to lift her back to the upright position and tuck her pillows in. As we did so, our fingers brushed, then pulled hastily apart. We avoided each other's eyes as the nurse straightened Mrs. L.'s nightie, tucked in her bedclothes, pulled the curtain back, and was gone as silently as she had appeared. I sat myself back down beside Mrs. Lovell as we recovered our collective breath. I loosened my itchy wool tie and slipped my top shirt button undone.

"Now, about these needles, Mrs. Lovell. Have they been taking fluid out of your tummy?"

“Lordie, yes, every time I’m in ’ere. Seems like it just keeps comin’ back. But I do feel ever so much better after they done it. Leastways, for a bit.”

Ascites! The word jumped into my head. What you get when your liver shuts down. Because of ... what was that thing called? Portal something … portal *hypertension*, that was it! That was why her stomach had been bleeding—all that back pressure. I felt like Sherlock Holmes and Doctor Watson all rolled into one, unscrambling a baffling whodunnit. Mrs. L. was drawing my attention to a scattering of marks on her arms and hands. Pinkish circles, four or five on each side, a spidery lacework extending outwards like tiny flowers.

“They’re allus peerin’ an’ pokin’ at these ’ere thingummies on me skin too, doc. Dunno ’ow long they been there.”

Oh, God, what were those called? Spider thingummies ... an inescapable sign of liver trouble. I could hardly wait to get at my *Cecil & Loeb*, become the world’s expert on liver failure before morning rounds. I love you, Mrs. L., I just love you. I’ll change your pussycat’s litter box anytime.

As I scooted out into the corridor heading for the library, I almost ran into my nurse chaperone. She was holding a sizeable tower of bed pans, which did nothing to lessen her beauty. I made a clumsy attempt to hold the door open for her. She paused to confront me.

“Look, I know Mrs. Lovell is a *good case* for the professor’s rounds. But you might not have shown such conspicuous delight at figuring what’s wrong with the poor woman. She might well not make it in next time she has a bleed.”

I stood there chastened as she swept past me and disappeared into the ward.

Origin of an Epidemic

Rare Cancer Seen in 41 Homosexuals.

Lawrence K. Altman, New York Times, July 3, 1981

Soon after I moved to the University of Florida in Gainesville, my department chairman urged me to sit for my pediatric hematology-oncology boards. Over the past eight years in London and Glasgow I had cared almost exclusively for children with cancer, so the hematology part was an almost closed book to me. In my position as an associate professor, I would often flounder on rounds with the residents and med students over questions like, "What does this thirteen-year-old's low hemoglobin mean?" "Can the surgeons operate on this baby with a longish bleeding time?" "Why does my patient with rheumatoid arthritis have a high white count?" I had rarely addressed any of these purely hematological issues but I was all too aware that the buck stopped with me.

When it came to requests for consultation from faculty members in other specialties, I would sneak peeks at the comprehensive reports of my immediate colleagues, who had all gone through three-year fellowships during their training and become well immersed in all things hematological. My own scribblings on the other hand lacked anything you could call definitive recommendations. To add to my anxiety, my new colleague, Paulette Mehta, let me know that a member of the examining board—Harvard's distinguished hematologist, David Nathan—had taken issue with the heavy bias towards oncology in the test questions, and had made sure this imbalance was addressed in full.

"Expect plenty of thorny questions on abstruse hematological issues affecting children," Paulette warned me. There was nothing for it but to bone up on my pitiful knowledge of the subject, so I started joining her in her hemophilia clinic. Paulette had for many years supervised the care of these boys with hemophilia, whereas my sole acquaintance with them had been during residency in London, when they would appear in Emergency at all hours, in dire need of fresh frozen plasma (FFP) infusions for a bleed into a knee or an ankle, or for an intractable nose bleed. If put to the test—as I would be all too soon—I could tell you that hemophilia comes mostly in two forms, and that it's caused by the inherited absence of either Factor VIII or IX in the affected person's plasma. Being genetically sex-linked it almost always affects boys, but that was the total sum of my knowledge.

I dimly recalled as a teenager making a house call with my doctor-uncle Ken to meet a middle-aged man with severe hemophilia. He had been confined to a wheelchair for most of his adult years, with his limb joints locked in one position from a lifetime of internal bleeding. So from the 1950s on, the regular infusion of donated FFP—rich in factor VIII and IX—to arrest these horrid hemorrhages had been greeted with jubilation by affected patients and their physicians alike. By the late 1960s, the concentrated form—cryoprecipitate (*cryo*)—had largely replaced FFP for the much commoner Factor VIII deficiency.

In 1981, three months into my new position at UF, I read an article in the *New York Times* that Sam Gross, our division chief, had passed on to us.

Rare Cancer Seen in 41 Homosexuals. Lawrence K. Altman, July 3, 1981

Doctors in New York and California have diagnosed among homosexual men 41 cases of a rare and often rapidly fatal form of cancer. Eight of the victims died less than 24 months after the diagnosis was made. The cause of the outbreak is unknown, and there is as yet no evidence of contagion. But the doctors who have made the diagnoses, mostly in New York City and the San Francisco Bay area, are alerting other physicians who treat large numbers of homosexual men to the problem, in an effort to help identify more cases and to reduce the delay in offering chemotherapy treatment.

None of us knew it at the time, but we were looking at the very first description of what became widely known as Acquired Immunodeficiency Syndrome (AIDS), manifesting itself in the form of the cancerous Kaposi's sarcoma.

"I don't know much about homosexuals in Florida," Sam commented, "but what I do know is that a lot of these guys are regular blood donors at Pheresis Centers, where they get paid. And we've got one downtown. Bad news for our hemophiliacs, because the CDC guys think this may be some kind of weird infection from their plasma."

"So you mean all our hemophiliacs run a risk every time we treat them?"

"Sure looks like it."

The next day I met ten-year-old Gary in Paulette's clinic. He had been needing frequent *cryo* infusions for swollen knees and ankles after trivial injuries, and he had been admitted the week before for bleeding that started under his tongue. It proved so hard to control that it threatened to obstruct his breathing. The idea of performing a tracheostomy to keep his airway open was too awful to contemplate, but that threat was ultimately averted with continuous *cryo* infusions for twenty-four hours.

I introduced myself to Gary and his mom. "I'm helping out Dr. Mehta today. I don't get to meet many guys like you, and I wanted to know more about how things are going with you all. Did you get back to school yet, Gary?"

"No, I've been sick. Fevers and stuff."

"I'm really worried about him, Doctor," his mother added. "He didn't have a temperature when we checked into the clinic, but it's up most evenings, and all his muscles ache, and he can't keep anything down."

I didn't find much amiss when I examined him, but he looked sick and I suspected his liver was a bit too big.

"Gary, I'm just going to chat with Dr. Mehta a minute. She knows you much better, so I want her to take a look at you too. Okay?"

He looked relieved, and I didn't blame him. Paulette had been looking after him since he was first diagnosed as an infant. I could almost hear Gary thinking,

What does this new guy know about anything? He wasn't too wide of the mark, though I had recently read about Hepatitis C showing up more often than expected in people getting frequent plasma infusions.

"Mom, Gary, I think we should run a few tests," Paulette said after she had finished her own exam. "We've been seeing a few odd infections in some of our boys, but it may be nothing at all to worry about."

A week later, Gary's results came back: tests for Hepatitis C were strongly positive. But before we could begin treatment the little guy was overtaken by a far worse fate. He started having trouble breathing, which got rapidly worse. Despite being rushed to our ICU, Gary succumbed to overwhelming pneumonia in both his lungs. The parents generously gave permission for an autopsy, which identified the cause of his rapid demise: *pneumocystis carinii*, a fungal infection that we knew especially affected people with weakened immunity.

"Some of those gay guys are getting the same thing," Sam said when we gathered to talk about the situation.

"And I've just got a positive Hep C test back on another of my hemophiliac boys," Paulette added. "It has to be linked to the *cryo* infusions. I'm going to have our infectious disease docs screen all of them, check what shape their immune systems are in."

It turned out that many of the boys had dangerously low levels of T-lymphocytes in their circulation—those cells derived from our thymus—putting them at risk for the same opportunistic infections affecting cancer patients on chemotherapy. It would be another two years before a virus would be isolated in both US and French labouratories that was almost certainly the cause of AIDS. But we soon established that the human immunodeficiency virus (HIV) was affecting many hemophiliacs including our own. We began to reserve *cryo* for particularly severe bleeds, and to only draw on Shands Hospital's pool of tried and tested donors.

Then Paulette got more bad news. “The education board is keeping two of our boys with Hep C out of school. Just when they’re gearing up for the new semester.”

“But they aren’t a risk to other children, are they?” I queried.

“Absolutely not. And I don’t think many of them will make it through their teens. So why have them just wait for the other shoe to drop?”

“Well, I’m going to take them to court,” Sam announced. “Get those boys back in school.”

The case was heard at the local courts, but the judge upheld the education board’s case, deciding there wasn’t enough evidence that the children posed no risk to others. Sam persuaded his lawyer to appeal, and the case was reheard in Tallahassee, the state’s capital. The appeals judge overturned the initial verdict, ruling that the education board must let these boys back in school, “effective immediately.” Any other children with complications thought to arise from their treatment must also be allowed normal schooling, “if they were considered by their treating physicians to be healthy enough to benefit from schooling, without risk either to themselves or other children.”

Sam celebrated by inviting us all to his house that Friday night, where the wine and beer flowed freely. But it was a hollow victory. In short order, several more boys succumbed to severe infections, including three more from pneumocystis pneumonia. Ultimately, none of Paulette’s band of hemophiliac boys survived to graduate from high school.

But by guess and by gosh, I somehow scraped through my pediatric hematology-oncology boards.

Hazards of Healthcare

When Jake started bleeding into his lungs, I quickly realized that I didn't know either him or his mother well enough to ask: "How hard do you want us to try here?" And this was far from the ideal time to start asking these kinds of questions.

We had been treating this hefty thirteen-year-old for a fast-growing brain tumour with chemotherapy drugs that had left him way short of all the normal cells in his circulation—the anticipated effect of such treatment. His platelets—the sticky guys that stop up your holes when you start bleeding—were in particularly short supply. We had been giving him transfusions of donated platelets at least once a day all this past week, but his body wasn't holding onto them for more than a few hours, and our blood bank was having to scour the country for good matches for his blood. Jake's resistance to all our treatments—it often took several staff to hold him down—might have warned me to expect trouble.

His blood pressure had been climbing all the last evening and through the early night hours, strongly suggesting a build-up of pressure inside his head. Now he was coughing up pink frothy blood in great gobs. It was four in the morning, and it seemed pretty clear that Jake wasn't long for this world. He himself was hastening this almost certain outcome by beating off all our efforts to give him extra oxygen, let alone pass an endotracheal tube into his windpipe to take over his breathing for him and get enough oxygen into his failing lungs.

"Let me f … ing die! I'm not your f … ing sweetheart!" was his croaking response to our combined efforts, between choking coughs that were bringing up massive bloody globs.

Too right, you're not, I found myself thinking, but kept the thought to myself. I realized I'd resorted to the word 'sweetheart' as I had tried to talk him down from his maddened struggles. I'm given to such words of endearment in times of stress; sometimes they can add a little warmth, even humour, to a grim scenario—but definitely not in Jake's case. His mother had insisted on staying right by Jake's side throughout this whole debacle and taken to cursing us out with a stream of *f ... ing a ... holes*—which certainly added to our futile efforts to resuscitate her son. The resident doctor, three nurses and I struggled between us to strap an oxygen mask in place on Jake's face, while simultaneously grabbing his flailing arms and trying to tie them down. One of the younger nurses had already taken a powerful blow to the head and had retreated in tears. The five of us who remained in the fray were now half-lying, half-sitting on his massive legs and feet, not unlike a police squad trying to apprehend a dangerous fugitive.

There was absolutely no room for more helpers. The confined space had become dammed up with people, with the machinery of life preservation, and with medical clutter of all kinds. The floor was awash with used and dropped syringes and plastic bags leaking various solutions, causing us to slip and slide in several directions as we grappled with a multitude of tasks. Blood from Jake's lungs, as well as from his blood vessels where catheters had become detached, had stained the morsels of paper on which someone had managed to scrawl records of his pulse and blood pressure and oxygen level, along with doses and times of the myriad drugs we had already decanted into his bloodstream. A cacophony of voices was raised as orders were bawled back and forth and test results were called in from the nearby emergency laboratory. It was abundantly evident from Jake's increasingly incoherent cursing and fighting us off that all our efforts were being conducted against this dying boy's will.

There was probably not a single member of the staff on the unit who wasn't involved in some way or another. Certainly no one was back in the nurses' changing room at the end of the corridor right next door to the family room. It had been left unlocked, we figured out later, so whoever had slipped inside at some point during the night had had the place to themselves. Shortly after we called off our final futile effort at resuscitation, and Jake's battered body had made its journey down four floors to the basement where hospital morgues are always located, we discovered that three credit cards, a check book, and fifty dollars in cash, had vanished from a student nurse's wallet.

There wasn't much time to speculate on this latest turn of events. Jake's mother had been threatening me pretty freely over the last few days: "If he dies, we'll be coming after you!" Not too subtle. I had never met any of Jake's family except his mother and grandmother but judging by the horde of visitors streaming in over the last few days, they had an extended family. The word must have gone out in the past forty-eight hours that something bad was going down with one of their own up at the university hospital. At one point the day before I had come across about a dozen people in the family room: several elders, a trio of diapered infants, and others of assorted ages in between. They had been talking heatedly among themselves when I stopped in, and I felt like an intruder in this hospital unit I was nominally in charge of. All my attempts to make acquaintance and fill them in on what was going on were met with stares and stony silence.

Once it was clear that there was nothing more to be done and I could leave the unit, I slipped downstairs to the Security Station on the hospital's first floor. I was greeted by Jackie's smiling face—an immensely welcome sight. A powerful and handsome black woman, Jackie had been maintaining law and order around here for as long as I could remember. I told her about the threats I had been receiving, and the final tragic outcome.

"You'd best take them to heart, Doc," she told me somberly after hearing me out. "But you can be sure we'll take good care of you!"

I found her words disquieting and comforting at once. After the strain of the last few hours, I was more than ready to be taken care of, but I restrained myself from curling up in her lap for a good bawl. True to her promise, no sooner had Jake's body been shipped off to the local funeral parlour than she appeared on the unit with two imposing henchmen to escort me off the premises. I knew I was secure in their company, and they didn't leave my side until I was safely in my car and pulling out of the parking lot. The image of police and criminals came to me once more, but this time I felt myself like the felon being carted off to jail.

"Stay away from campus until things quiet down," Jackie counseled me. "Stay out of the stores and the mall. Don't answer your phone, but I want you to check in with me every day."

It put me in mind of a colleague of mine—another pediatric oncologist in Fort Worth, Texas. Something even more frightening had happened to him during his training fellowship ten years before at St Jude's, the Memphis hospital dedicated to children's cancer research and treatment. The father of a boy who had died of leukemia kept my friend, plus a nurse and a ward clerk, at gunpoint in an office on one of the hospital units for thirty-six hours. They were rescued only by a police SWAT team bursting in and fatally wounding the bereaved father.

My enforced vacation felt like police protection extended to one who has turned evidence to the Feds against the Mafia. Jake's extended family took itself back home to lick its wounds and mourn its lost son. But not before each one of them had been frisked down by Security, which yielded the haul of an unloaded pistol and a carving knife. I had plenty of time over the next week to reflect on the rights and wrongs of our actions that night. Perhaps we tried too hard in what I had known from the start was a futile attempt to save Jake's life. The family had done its best to intimidate me, but his underlying cancer had already shown almost no signs of responding to any of our treatments, and I had done my best to let the family know how slim his chances were. Jake himself had also made it crystal clear that he had had enough.

I never heard any more from his folks, and I don't know if my letter of condolence ever reached them. The next Monday I was back at work, though it took me a long and spooky time to stop looking over my shoulder as I walked a lonely hospital corridor at night.

Twins

Renee had a school project. Her seventh-grade class had been set the task of composing an essay on some aspect of American society. She had settled on tackling the health care system, and after some thought had decided—perhaps her mother had a part in this—to come and interview me.

It was five years since I had last seen Renee, having decided at that final clinic visit that I didn't need to make more routine follow-up appointments. The family lived in town and her father was on the neurosurgery faculty of our medical school. We would pass each other on the stairs every six months or so or find ourselves in the same line for a cup of coffee, and he would update me on Renee's exploits. This seemed as good a way of checking on her as bringing her back into my clinic. I knew full well that her mother would be in touch with me soon enough, should anything at all out of line happen to their remaining daughter.

Renee started to quiz me, shuffling the three pieces of foolscap paper she had laid out on her knees. She'd prepared her questions well.

"Why did you become a doctor? Why a pediatrician? Why an oncologist?"

She pronounced the words precisely: a serious child wise beyond her thirteen years. We were sitting in tall rocking chairs that faced each other four feet apart in the rear of unit 94B's nursing station. Her presence there with me on the children's oncology ward took me back a decade. Did she have any memory, I wondered, of all those days and nights she and her mother had spent here?

She went on tossing out her fearless questions. "Where did you go to school? Do you have children? What do you like to do when you're not working?"

I caught myself mulling over what her seventh-grade teacher would make of reading my personal story in this term paper on American health care. It seemed like it might come to look more like a college admission essay.

Renee was already a couple of inches taller than her mother, who stood silent and still behind her chair. When her mother had called me on the phone to set things up, she had told me with rare candour that she would sometimes in her dreams hear my tread down our Cancer Center corridor. She would wait for the pause beside each exam room door, which signalled the verdict on her daughter's blood count. The judgment that would tell her if this one too was to be taken from her. It was something about the length of the pause, she told me, that signalled to her if the news was good or bad.

I had first met the family twelve years earlier when the twins were just over twelve months old. Renee was diagnosed with acute leukemia in late February, on my birthday. A month later to the day, her sister Lise came down with the same thing. Two cases of leukemia in identical twins are not so unusual, though there is no such tendency when twins are non-identical. We still know precious little about the causes of this disease in children, but there has to be a clue here. Perhaps there are faulty genes that don't know to put up a fight when a cancer cell starts to lay its eggs in their happy home. Or some cancer-causing virus gets inside this single embryo at a critical time in the pregnancy and stealthily prepares a nest in which the foreign cells may grow. But what virus? Which gene? Therein lies the mystery.

The twins responded the way almost all young girls with leukemia respond to their initial chemotherapy. Within a month of diagnosis, Lise had followed Renee into a state of what we call remission. There was not a trace of cancer to be seen in either of them. Pediatric oncologists learned decades ago, though, not to equate this situation with cure. The leukemia cells had simply gone underground, and a long war of attrition was just getting underway to root them out for good.

When identical twins are both affected—and it usually happens early in their lives—the leukemia looks and behaves very much alike in the two of them. At least that's the rule of thumb. Trying to offer some comfort to her parents after Lise first became ill, I told them they had every reason for hope. Young girls with leukemia seem to respond better than older children. Renee was already showing all the signs of continuing to do fine with her treatments, and that there was no reason to think Lise wouldn't follow suit.

So much for rules of thumb—it was not to work out that way. Renee, the first to go down with the disease, never looked back once her treatment got underway. She stayed in almost blooming health throughout her three years of prescribed therapy and, as was abundantly clear when she came to interview me, she was continuing to thrive more than a decade later. But Lise's state of temporary remission was to last less than six months. Then the leukemia exploded again in full force within her. With more intensive treatment she achieved another shaky hold on things, which kept her going for another eight months. After that, the cancer gathered its forces and took her life, just fifteen months after it had first made its presence known within her.

Ten years on, her mother was still haunted by what I had told her that first day. The day we diagnosed her second daughter, she was emerging from a sleepless night at Renee's bedside. Renee had just come through her first month of chemotherapy. She was looking down the road at three more years of in-and-out-of-hospital stays, interspersed with weekly clinic visits. I had sought to lift her spirits a little, quoting the medical literature that told us that Lise's odds were every bit as good, and that, like Renee, she had at least a two-to-one chance of surviving and thriving.

"Little girls make up the largest group of those who seem to be cured of their leukemia," I added, "and your two have everything going for them."

Within a year I was eating my words. Once the course of the girls' leukemia, and their lives, abruptly diverged, I suspect their mother put no further stock in medical statistics. Or in me, perhaps. I could hardly blame her, especially because I could offer her no good reason for the disparity. If she doubted my competence to care for her remaining daughter, she was too courteous, or too reserved in both emotion and judgment, ever to express such thoughts. But it seems her dread of Renee's monthly blood counts never left her dreams.

Ten years on, her surviving daughter was continuing to ply me with her carefully rehearsed questions. I started to loop my own back to her:

"Do you remember me? The hospital? All those shots?"

"Yes," was all she said, this solemn young woman, her mother's daughter in every way. "Yes, I remember you."

What feelings were hidden behind her steadfast gaze I had no way of discerning. Then I ventured the question that was beating away inside my chest.

"And your sister Lise? Do you remember her?"

"Yes, I remember her."

She said nothing more. Her mother stayed mute behind her chair, her eyes down, fixed on a point on the top of her daughter's head. One question I held back, left forever unasked, and unanswered: *Why was it that Lise, your twin, was taken? And why do you, Renee, remain here, a young woman in such glowing health, to question me for your school project?*

Recently, a friend of both mine and of this family offered me a postscript to this story. Renee, now seventeen, was at a local beach celebrating the Fourth of July. My friend was married to one of our university faculty and several faculty families had made this an annual outing. The teenagers were toweling off after bathing when they heard frantic shouts from some way out in the ocean. A young boy had been swept out to sea and was in obvious danger of not making it back to shore. Without pausing, Renee tossed her towel aside, plunged back into the sea, and within a few dozen strong strokes was able to reach the boy and haul him to safety.

If you believe in *karma*, you'll know that I had the answer to my unasked question.

The Sign

One Saturday afternoon I was sitting with the parents and siblings of a five-month-old baby who had stopped breathing an hour earlier. Eddie had had leukemia from birth, and I met him and his parents on his first day of life after their obstetrician had spotted multiple small blue and red lumps over his face and trunk.

"I've never seen anything like this before," the obstetrician had told Eddie's mom and dad, Rose and Sam, gently. "I think we should get him to the university hospital right away, so they can find out what this is all about."

I got called to the Emergency Room after the residents noted that Eddie also had a large liver and spleen, and a blood test had shown a high white blood cell count and low platelets, all suggesting leukemia. The following morning our pediatric surgeon biopsied one of the larger nodules in the operating room, and I collected a bone marrow sample. Both confirmed the presence of acute myeloblastic leukemia, the less common and more aggressive form of leukemia that affects children. This was the first time in twenty years as a pediatric oncologist that I had seen a newborn with congenital leukemia. I scanned what I could find in the literature—and it proved pretty sparse.

With Rose and Sam's agreement we did what seemed to be the best thing—that is, to start Eddie on our standard protocol of chemotherapy for his type of leukemia. But after two courses of drugs, which made him horribly sick, Eddie had had only a partial and brief response in both his blood and skin lesions. Switching our drug regimen proved equally futile, and when the tiny child developed bilateral pneumonia, it seemed to all his caregivers to be a blessing.

Sam, Eddie's father, was just back from thirty hours on his routine truck route up to Knoxville, Tennessee, and back. Arriving at the pediatric intensive care unit, he took in the scene, heard me out about how we expected Eddie to die any moment, then called his four elder children to join him and his wife and me in the social worker's room.

"Eddie was just visiting with us here, checking out how we were doing as a family," he told his children. "Now he's going back to Heaven."

His older children looked at him wide-eyed. There was a long pause before anyone said anything. Then Rose, Eddie's mother, broke the silence: "No. No, not yet. I need a sign." Sam looked set to press his case, but he held back whatever he was about to add, instead closed his eyes as though in prayer. Then: "I understand, Rose. We'll wait on a sign." All six family members closed their eyes for another long moment.

There was no alternative. The ICU staff got ready to intubate the baby and hook him up to a ventilator. Normally a routine enough procedure in this unit, but it took more brute force than skill to get the endotracheal tube in place and inflate Eddie's congested little lungs with a sufficient supply of oxygen. An hour later in the grocery store aisle I got an urgent page.

"The tube's out, John," the ICU nurse yelled down the phone, startling several of my fellow shoppers. "It's bedlam, we can't get Rose calmed down enough to decide if she wants us to keep on trying. Get here as soon as you can, will you?"

By the time I arrived back in Eddie's pod, everybody was once more embarked on the bloody business of getting another breathing tube down Eddie's tiny trachea. Rose insisted on staying right beside his crib, which wasn't helping matters. But as soon as she saw me, she flung herself on me and moaned, "Stop! It's okay. It's the sign!"

"Are you sure now, Rose? It looks like they just got the tube back in place again."

"I'm sure. It's the sign. You don't have to go on. But…" she was crying freely but managed to draw in a long breath. "I want my mom and dad here. And my sister."

“Of course. We’ll wait on them.”

What I had not taken into account was that the final whistle had just blown on a home game at “The Swamp”—the Florida Gators’ football stadium. The stadium was less than a quarter mile from the hospital, and ninety-thousand spectators were at that moment pouring out of the stadium into the surrounding streets. Somehow the PICU staff managed to keep Eddie alive on the ventilator for a full six hours, which was how long it took for Rose’s parents and sister to make it to the hospital.

We finally gathered in a semicircle as the ICU attending doctor prepared to remove the endotracheal tube—this time deliberately and for good. Rose never wavered again in her decision and mostly sat quietly waiting with Sam and the other children. One of the resident doctors injected a large dose of Fentanyl into Eddie’s IV line to make sure the baby would be quite unaware of what was happening. As the senior doctor gradually drew the tube out from the infant’s trachea, he gasped just once before his whole body began to darken. I could still hear his heartbeat for a minute, maybe a little longer, before it finally stopped and never beat again.

Between them Rose and Sam gathered Eddie up into Rose’s arms, murmured to him and stroked his head as the whole family gathered around her. Rose cried a few more tears, then looked around at us caregivers. She broke into a big beam.

“Why don’t y’all hold him?”

Taking her cue, we permitted ourselves a collective smile. I stepped up to take Eddie from his mom, then passed him to the nurse next to me And so it went for several minutes. Later, I reflected on what had been in the end a good death. It seems there has to be some purpose in such a happening, to such a short and tragic life as Eddie’s. All I remember is all the hugging, the tears, the laughter, then more hugging. I have never before or since hugged so many fellow workers. For a short time, our intensive care unit was transformed into a sacred place of community. Of communion.

Epilogue

Attention, taken to its highest degree, is the same thing as prayer

Simone Weil

To pay attention, this is our endless and proper work

Mary Oliver

I started out reflecting on the nature of healing. I reminded myself, and perhaps you, that healing is an intransitive verb. Patients do their own healing, although we doctors and nurses and others hopefully lend a hand. In these stories of my own journeys, my part has been that of a supportive witness more than a direct agent of healing. And throughout my almost fifty years in medicine I have been on my own self-healing journey—though I was not always aware of it.

As I sit at my computer in my upstairs office, I can turn my head a few inches to the left and gaze at my mother's beautiful face. It is a photo of Mummy as a young adult in the early 1930's. She is dressed in what looks like a flapper dress, as though she were about to dance the Charleston. She has now been dead almost seventy years, and I ended my earlier memoir, *Journeys with a Thousand Heroes*, with the letter I wrote to her. I thanked her for the greatest gift she had bestowed on me: that of being fully *present* until her death when I was twelve years old. This is the most holistic form of care there can be. It took me a working lifetime to recognize it was my mother who taught me the capacity for *attention*—for being present in body, mind, and spirit to those who came to me in need.

The word *servant* comes from the Greek, θεραπς (theraps), from which we get *therapist*. But servant also means *attendant*, and nowadays that label gets attached to us doctors—the *attending* physician. "Attention is prayer," said the

French mystic and philosopher Simone Weil. And the Pulitzer Prize-winning poet Mary Oliver says in her poem, *Yes! No!*, "Imagination is better than a sharp instrument. To pay attention, this is our endless and proper work." To my mind, the best attending doctors are those who bring to their work what Tibetan Buddhists call compassionate objectivity, especially in their care of dying patients.

Being a Quaker has given me belief in spirit medicine. Children are often more in touch with their spiritual selves than we grown-ups, perhaps especially when life-limiting illness confronts them. Late in my career, I became medical director of a children's hospice. I visited my patients in their homes and was often present at their bedsides when they died. When three-year-old Marie came home for the last time, she didn't want to sleep in her bedroom anymore. She was scared of something, her mom told me, though her daughter couldn't articulate what was bothering her. Her parents made up a comfy mattress-bed on the living room floor and took turns sleeping beside her, so that Marie had one of them close to her all the time. Then on the evening of her death, she announced:

"Mommy, I want to go back in my own room. I want to play with my friends."

Within minutes of being tucked up in her own bed for the first time in several weeks, Marie closed her eyes and slipped away. We were left to ponder the comforting mystery of who those friends of hers might be.

The opportunity to draw so close to another always offers a healing experience for both. Quite wonderful that it is never a one-way street. I used to speculate how often other medical colleagues encountered these kinds of feelings—what Louise Erdrich calls in her novel, *Love Medicine,* "the touch." Then I found myself at the annual conference of the American Holistic Medical Association. I was greeted at the door by a group of half-a-dozen doctors wearing multicoloured tee shirts with the logo *Hugs Heal* on the back. Those magical three days began with yoga and tai chi, healthy breakfasts, and invigorating walks: a conscious journey of *self-healing*. How come it had taken me most of my working life to discover these medical colleagues—to discover that I wasn't alone?

This led on to my meeting a group of physicians who were holding weekend gatherings to come to terms with the medical profession's cumulative sense of failure and grief. Throughout our training and practice our primary task is drummed into us: to cure every patient of every illness. This small group of like-minded doctors had come to realize that we would be a whole lot healthier if we could just free ourselves from such a notion. And that the only way to do so was to help each other shake ourselves free of these chronic feelings of inadequacy and failure.

I joined ten women and two other men for this weekend workshop at the Michigan home of one of the women, who led us in building enough trust in each other to freely share our vulnerabilities and sadness. In time we felt loosened up enough to cry in front of each other, which led in turn to a good deal of laughter. Just like at wakes—and perhaps that's what it was: a wake for those countless people who had come to us in need, and whom we could never restore to full health.

After supper on the first day, we gathered in a large huddle in front of an open fireplace in the living room to share happier stories of our lives and our families. Our hostess produced several large blankets and duvets and announced the sleeping arrangements. The ten women would snuggle for the night together in this room, while we men were to head upstairs to the single king-size bed. By this time, it seemed a perfectly okay arrangement for us three to be climbing under the covers together in our underwear. We chatted idly for only a short while longer before settling into delicious and dreamless sleep. Expressing our cumulative emotions so freely had clearly prepared us well for slumber.

I woke to the morning light in the intimate company of two other members of what I could now call the *self-healing* profession. This had been the first time in my life I had shared a bed with two other men. I've spent forty-seven years learning and practicing the science and art of caregiving. I've worked at four universities—London and Glasgow from 1960 to 1976, and Case Western and Florida from 1976 to 2007. In this final quarter of my life, I've embarked on a new adventure.

I've changed countries once more and am the proud holder of a Canadian passport to add to my British and American ones. I've spent my last fifteen years drawing UK and US retirement cheques while discovering the mosaic that is Canada—a tableau that blends not only Britain and America but every other country I know. I am blissfully married to my Canadian wife, Dorothy, whom I met in Gainesville during a three-week course we staged on art and healing. And I'm on a different kind of learning curve—though as steep in its way as my early years of doctoring. Our small publishing house, *HARP The People's Press* (www.harppublishing.ca), is dedicated to exploring the arts and how they can help us heal ourselves in body, mind and spirit. What further adventures await?

Acknowledgments

My grateful thanks to all who have helped me create *Healing by Intent*—reading drafts, offering constructive comments, and writing generous testimonials. I'm especially grateful to my editor, Troon Harrison, who guided me in countless ways to improve both the book's story and its style.

As a social enterprise, HARP works with many of our community's artists. I offer a special tribute to Sara Avmaat, who created the cover art, to digital designer Cathy Lin for the layout and design, to Gillian McCulloch for her skill as a portrait artist, and to social media maven Denise Davies for her help with promotion and countless other tasks.

Last and most enduring, my love and gratitude to the multitude of young people and their families I've been privileged to serve over close on half a century.

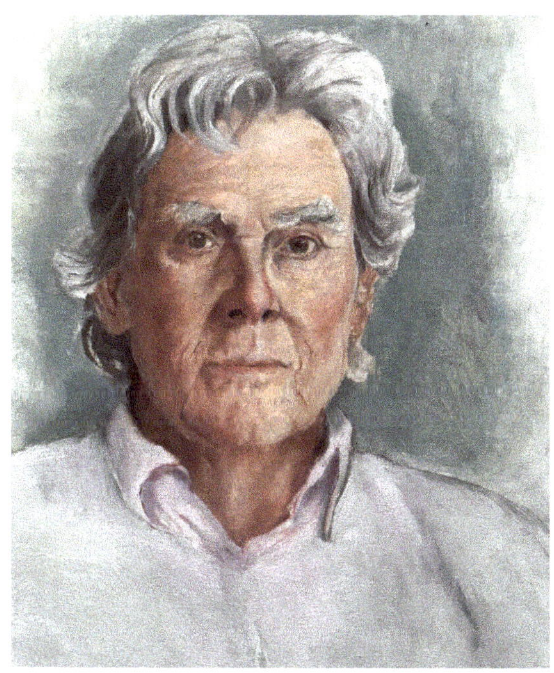

Portrait by Gillian McCulloch

John Graham-Pole is a retired professor of pediatrics. He has been a clinician, teacher, and pioneer researcher in the field of childhood cancer for forty years. Educated in Britain, he co-founded the Center for Arts in Medicine at the University of Florida, now among the world's leading arts-and-health organizations.

He is an author of eleven works of fiction, non-fiction, and poetry. He recently published *Songlines*, the third in a trilogy of novels inspired by young people he has known with cancer. He lives in Nova Scotia with his wife, Dorothy Lander, where they co-founded HARP: The People's Press (www.harppublishing.ca), a multimedia publishing house dedicated to exploring how the arts can enhance our individual and communal health. This is his second medical memoir—a follow-up to *Journeys with a Thousand Heroes.*

His personal website is www.johngrahampole.com and he can be found on Facebook and LinkedIn.

www.ingramcontent.com/pod-product-compliance
Ingram Content Group UK Ltd.
Pitfield, Milton Keynes, MK11 3LW, UK
UKHW021831270726
14058UKWH00001B/81

9 780993 829581